By Barry Meier

PAIN KILLER

MISSING MAN

SPOOKED

PAIN KILLER

PAIN KILLER

An Empire of Deceit and the Origin

of America's Opioid Epidemic

BARRY MEIER

Random House
New York

2023 Random House Trade Paperback Edition

Copyright © 2003, 2018 by Barry Meier

Published in the United States by Random House,
an imprint and division of Penguin Random House LLC, New York.

RANDOM HOUSE and the HOUSE colophon are registered trademarks
of Penguin Random House LLC.

Originally published in hardcover by Rodale,
an imprint of Random House,
a division of Penguin Random House LLC, in 2003.
The second edition of this work was published in hardcover
by Random House, an imprint and division of
Penguin Random House LLC, in 2018.

Library of Congress Cataloging-in-Publication Data

Names: Meier, Barry, author.
Title: Pain killer : an empire of deceit and the origin of
America's opioid epidemic / Barry Meier.
Description: 2nd edition. | New York : Random House, 2018. |
Includes bibliographical references and index.
Identifiers: LCCN 2018010496 | ISBN 9781984801180 |
ISBN 9780525511090 (ebook)
Subjects: | MESH: Opioid-Related Disorders—epidemiology |
Socioeconomic Factors | Oxycodone—history | Opioid-Related
Disorders—history | Drug Overdose—epidemiology | History,
20th Century | History, 21st Century | United States
Classification: LCC HV5822.O99 | NLM WM 286 | DDC 362.29/9—dc23
LC record available at lccn.loc.gov/2018010496

Printed in the United States of America on acid-free paper

randomhousebooks.com

2 4 6 8 9 7 5 3 1

Book design by Virginia Norey

CONTENTS

Book of the Dead

WITHIN A SPAN OF THIRTY-SIX HOURS IN PHILADELPHIA, NINE bodies had been found just blocks away from one another. Five were inside homes. Two were in cars. Two were on the street. The oldest of them was forty-two. The youngest was twenty-four.

They had names but they would soon become statistics, data points consumed by a tidal wave of fatal drug overdoses sweeping across the United States. In 2016, 64,000 Americans died from drug overdoses. That number equals the population of cities such as Portland, Maine; Lynchburg, Virginia; and Santa Fe, New Mexico. It was as if, in one year, a plague had entered one of these towns and killed every single inhabitant. It seemed like a horrible high-water mark, but the annual overdose death toll kept climbing and, by 2021, had topped 100,000, a jump of 56 percent in five years.

Bodies were piling up too fast in some places for medical examiners and coroners to keep up. Morgues were filled to capacity, and corpses had to be stored for days in rented refrigerated tractor-trailers until space became available. Many of the dead were not autopsied. It is standard procedure in a drug-overdose case to conduct an autopsy. But even if medical examiners had

had time to autopsy every victim, some stopped themselves from doing so. Professional groups that accredit medical examiners set a limit on the number of autopsies that a doctor can competently perform in a year, and examiners in areas with large numbers of overdose deaths would have exceeded that number and risked losing their accreditation. As a result, when overdose victims were discovered near hypodermic needles or pill bottles, they went straight to their graves, unexamined. The vast majority of these deaths involved "opioids," prescription painkillers or illegal drugs derived from compounds either found in the opium poppy or synthesized in a lab.

The opioid crisis has become woven into the fabric of everyday American life. In hospitals, newborns, separated from the narcotics coursing through the bloodstream of their addicted mothers, enter the world writhing in the pain of opioid withdrawal. On the streets, police officers carry a new piece of standard equipment, a nasal spray containing medicine that could save the life of a person in the midst of an overdose. The epidemic's impact has been so pervasive that life expectancy among white men in the United States has started falling for the first time in more than twenty years.

Public officials have called for a dramatic response. Lawmakers urged that tens of billions of dollars be spent to treat the addicted. Newspapers, magazines, and television programs are filled with reports about the havoc caused in communities large and small.

All this attention makes it seem as if something new is happening. That's not the case. The recent appearance of counterfeit versions of a particularly potent synthetic opioid, fentanyl, has driven up the body count. But by 2021, some 250,000 Americans had died during the two preceding decades from overdoses involving legal drugs that were produced by pharmaceutical companies and prescribed by doctors.

People have long been sounding alarms about the mounting death toll linked to prescription painkillers. Still, year after year, politicians, lawmakers, public regulators, professional medical organizations, and insurers have neglected the growing carnage while the pharmaceutical industry has downplayed it. The result is tragic and predictable. By 2021, the number of overdose deaths involving prescription opioids had quadrupled since 1999. A disaster that might have been contained with an early response had morphed into a hydra.

Every catastrophe, natural or man-made, has a beginning. For the opioid crisis, the seed was a drug called OxyContin. When OxyContin first appeared in the mid-1990s, it was heralded as a "wonder" drug that would change how pain, mankind's oldest and most persistent medical enemy, was treated. A determined band of activists laid the groundwork for its arrival by arguing that millions of people were suffering unnecessarily because doctors had exaggerated fears about the addictive potential of prescription painkillers. Doctors had used the term "narcotic" to describe the active ingredients in such medications. But advocates of more-aggressive pain treatment were so eager to distance drugs like OxyContin from the back-alley connotations of "narcotic" that they coined the word "opioid" to rebrand them.

OxyContin became the centerpiece of the most aggressive marketing campaign for a powerful and potentially addicting narcotic ever undertaken by the pharmaceutical industry. Its producer, Purdue Pharma, showered millions of dollars on doctors to convince them to prescribe OxyContin and claimed that it offered not only a better way to treat pain but a safer one as well. Purdue, which was owned by one of America's wealthiest and most secretive families, the Sacklers, would make billions from the drug's sales.

When this book was first published, in 2003, many of the critical events chronicled in this new and expanded edition had yet to take place. For instance, in 2007, Purdue and three of its top executives pled guilty to criminal charges in connection with the company's marketing of OxyContin.

With the case's end, I thought my involvement in the story was over. I also labored under the misconception, as journalists often do, that when one stops reporting on a story the story stops. Unfortunately, that has not proven to be the case. If anything, the OxyContin episode spawned an era of chaos, corporate profiteering, political entropy, and misery, some of which might have been prevented by federal officials. Following the plea agreements with Purdue and its officials, the Justice Department consigned to secrecy evidence its own investigators had uncovered about when Purdue first learned about OxyContin's abuse and what the company did with this crucial information. After a decade in obscurity, scores of internal Purdue emails and other records unearthed by investigators are finally available to shed new light on the origin story of the opioid crisis. OxyContin was not a "wonder" drug. It was the gateway drug to the most devastating public-health disaster of the twenty-first century.

PAIN KILLER

ONE

Pill Hill

LATE ON A JANUARY NIGHT IN 2000, THE TELEPHONE RANG IN the bedroom of a country doctor named Art Van Zee. He listened while a nurse at a nearby hospital explained that a young woman had just been brought into the emergency room after overdosing on a painkiller. She was in the intensive-care unit on a respirator.

It was Van Zee's night on call, so he eased out of bed, quietly dressed, and left the house. He drove down a long dirt driveway, past a man-made trout pond and a corral that was home to his children's ponies and donkeys. At the bottom of the driveway, he passed a small concrete building that served as his wife's law office and then turned right onto a two-lane highway that led from Dryden, Virginia, to Pennington Gap, a larger town and the location of Lee County Community Hospital.

Art Van Zee was fifty-two and had grown up thousands of miles away from this slice of Appalachia, in the small, high-desert city of Elko, Nevada. But after twenty-five years of living in Lee County, he had come to love everything about this place—its landscape, its culture, and its separateness—and it had embraced him as one of its own.

Lee County lies in southwestern Virginia, wedged between

Kentucky and Tennessee. It is a place of breathtaking beauty as well as intense poverty. The Cumberland Mountains run through its heart and, over time, fast-running streams have sliced from them steep stony mountain ridges, plunging hollows, and gentle valleys. Stands of loblolly pine, shortleaf pine, hickory, and oak rise out of the soil. Below the land are rich veins of coal, the source of Appalachia's wealth and its heartache. Just over the Kentucky border from Lee County is Harlan County, the scene of several violent mine-worker strikes, including the 1974 strike that became the subject of an Oscar-winning documentary, *Harlan County U.S.A.*

Art Van Zee had first come to Lee County that same year, as part of a contingent of Vanderbilt University medical students who traveled through Appalachia giving out free physical examinations. When he came back two years later, as a volunteer in a federal government program that sends doctors into poor areas that have few physicians, Van Zee took over a community health clinic in the small Lee County town of St. Charles.

St. Charles, which lies at the intersection of several small roads and railroad spurs, had once been an Appalachian boomtown, with a hotel, a bank, movie theaters, and restaurants. When Van Zee arrived in 1976, coal-digging machines had displaced miners and St. Charles was fast on its way to becoming a ghost town. Mining was still part of the region. Scores of miners and their families continued to live in hardscrabble coal camps, collections of shacks, tar-paper shanties, and broken-down homes that lined the roads leading to the mines. At regular intervals, a screeching sound, like the scrape of a giant piece of chalk against a blackboard, echoed near mines that were still operating. It was the squeal of iron wheels against railway tracks, as a locomotive slowly eased container cars under a hopper so they could be loaded with coal.

Van Zee, tall and gangly with a salt-and-pepper beard, could have practiced anywhere. But his father was a Presbyterian minister who had instilled in him the notion that work should be a form of service. So Van Zee performed his work in Lee County, where medical services were painfully scarce, with a missionary's intensity. He organized smoking-cessation contests. He brought in experts to perform cancer screenings. He ran fairs that offered prenatal care. He even put together courses on healthier cooking, a hard sell in a part of the country where anything edible runs the risk of being fried. Each year, thousands of people passed through the St. Charles clinic and were treated for every imaginable illness. For those too sick to come in, Van Zee made house calls, driving out to coal camps. When mining disasters struck, he stood by the mouth of the pits even when the only help he could give was to those recovering bodies. His was an all-consuming job. One night, his car was found blocking traffic. He was in the driver's seat, passed out from exhaustion while waiting for a red light to change.

On this January night, it took Van Zee about fifteen minutes to reach Lee County Hospital, a small but modern facility. The young woman, he was told, had overdosed on a narcotic painkiller called OxyContin. She had been visiting her parents when she fell out of bed with such a thump that they raced into her room. They found her lying on the floor, comatose and close to death. Narcotics depress the respiratory system, and most fatalities involving them occur because people stop breathing. To revive the woman, hospital physicians had put an emergency breathing tube down her throat and connected it to a respirator.

At the time, Van Zee had little experience with OxyContin. In 2000, the medication was relatively new to the marketplace, and he knew only that it was a time-release painkiller in the same class of drugs as morphine. He had prescribed it only a few times, to patients suffering from cancer or those who had undergone numerous surgeries for back pain without finding relief.

Van Zee knew just about everybody in Lee County, but the respirator's mask obscured the patient's face. He picked up her chart and saw her name. Twenty-one years earlier, he had held her as a three-month-old baby and given her immunization shots. Since then, he had treated her for childhood illnesses and watched her grow into a thriving teenager.

He took a deep breath. In recent months, both a local drug-abuse counselor and a druggist in Pennington Gap had told Van Zee that OxyContin had started to show up for sale on the street. Van Zee hadn't paid much attention to their concerns. He had always been conservative when it came to prescribing drugs, and it never would have occurred to him that not all doctors were as scrupulous as he was. He and other adults in Pennington Gap also had yet to realize what area teenagers already knew: that a tablet of OxyContin, or Oxy, as the drug was called, was the ticket to a great high.

One of those teenagers, Lindsay Myers, had first tried the drug in the spring of 1999 when she was sixteen, and she took a certain pride in being among the youngest Oxy users she knew. She was a sophomore at Lee County High School, a cheerleader for Lee High's football team, the Generals, and a runner. Lindsay had a round, pretty face, and her brown eyes were offset by dark-blond hair, which she pulled back into a ponytail. She was the kind of girl that boys noticed, and she came from one of the wealthiest families in the area. Her mother's father had founded a company that operated coal mines in Kentucky and Virginia, and Lindsay's father, Johnny, had joined the family business. While most kids at Lee High walked to school or were lucky to drive hand-me-down cars, she tooled around in a brand-new black Jeep Cherokee. It was a far better car than her teachers could afford.

Overlooking Pennington Gap, a town of 1,800, was the Myers family's large, modern house, which appeared more like an upper-class dwelling in suburban Atlanta than a home in small-town Appalachia. Lindsay wished she lived in Atlanta, a seven-hour drive to the south. She loved visiting the city on shopping trips with her mother, Jane, or going there with friends to attend rock concerts. Like most teenagers in Pennington Gap, she felt bored. There wasn't much to do, see, or buy. The city's tiny downtown, two blocks straddling railroad tracks, had only a few stores. The main clothing store, Gibson's, displayed dresses that a teenager would have never bought.

Most of Pennington Gap's action took place at its east end, where a two-lane road entered the town. Fast-food restaurants clustered near the intersection. Kids from Lee High liked to hang out at McDonald's, but Lindsay went to Hardee's, which attracted a slightly older crowd of people in their early or mid-twenties. They threw better parties and had drugs, or knew where to get them.

She first tried Oxy while riding around in a car outside Pennington Gap. Lindsay watched a friend pop a small blue tablet into his mouth and let it sit there for a few minutes before taking it out and wiping it on his T-shirt. He then dropped it into a creased dollar bill and folded the bill into a tight envelope. Putting the packet into his mouth, he bit down hard on it and then dumped the crushed powder onto a plastic compact-disc holder. Lindsay snorted some of it.

She didn't get high that first time, but friends kept raving about OxyContin, and a girlfriend told her about someone dealing Oxys in Harlan, Kentucky, a thirty-minute drive from Pennington Gap. The two girls took off in Lindsay's Jeep and found the address they were looking for. They stopped the car in front of a darkened house. Lindsay handed her friend $150 and waited until she came back with four pills. On the drive home, they pulled off the road, crushed up the pills, and snorted them.

At first, Lindsay felt sick to her stomach. But the nausea quickly passed and a rush of warmth spread through her body as her muscles relaxed. Every tension, every care evaporated. Nothing else had made her feel that way. Back in Pennington Gap, the two girls cruised the main drag for a while. Then Lindsay started feeling sleepy. By the time she got home, she couldn't keep her eyes open and was soon wrapped in a delicious cocoon of sleep.

The recreational use of prescription painkillers was nothing new, either in Lee County or in many other parts of the United States. For decades, some patients and drug abusers had misused popular painkillers sold under names such as Percocet, Percodan, and Tylox. The active ingredient in those drugs is a narcotic called oxycodone, and each pill typically contained 5 milligrams of oxycodone mixed with 500 milligrams of an over-the-counter pain reliever such as aspirin or acetaminophen.

OxyContin was very different. It was pure oxycodone, and the weakest dosage contained 10 milligrams of the narcotic, twice as much as in its predecessors. It was also available in much higher dosages, including 20, 40, 80, and 160 milligrams of oxycodone. In terms of pure narcotic firepower, OxyContin was a nuclear weapon.

The drug was first marketed in 1996 by a little-known Connecticut company named Purdue Pharma. To produce OxyContin, Purdue used a patented time-release formula that allowed the company to pack large amounts of oxycodone into the drug. The tablet's narcotic payload was released gradually, some reaching the patient's bloodstream within the first hour, and the remainder over the following eleven hours.

OxyContin's time-release design ("contin" was short for "continuous") gave it an edge over older painkillers such as Percocet and Tylox. Patients felt the result of those drugs faster, but they only provided relief for four hours, and a pain sufferer might have to wake up in the middle of the night to take another pill. But Purdue Pharma also claimed that OxyContin would be less appealing than traditional painkillers to drug abusers. Addiction experts have long known that people who abuse drugs are drawn to a drug based on its strength and the speed at which its effect is felt. So it wasn't unreasonable to theorize that OxyContin, with its time-release design, wouldn't give drug abusers a quick high. It didn't take long, however, for even novice abusers like Lindsay Myers to discover that an OxyContin tablet, softened up with a little water or saliva, could be crushed to yield its oversize narcotic payload all at once.

Before long, Lindsay was scoring one or two Oxys a day. The Drug Enforcement Administration (DEA), the federal agency that polices the manufacture, shipping, and dispensing of prescription drugs, had placed OxyContin within the most tightly controlled category of medications, so-called Schedule II narcotics. OxyContin's classmates in Schedule II included such other powerful and potentially addictive painkillers as morphine, Dilaudid, and fentanyl. Under federal law, every gram of these substances is supposed to be tracked and accounted for as it moves from manufacturer to distributor and from distributor to doctor or druggist. Lindsay bought most of her pills from a woman nicknamed "Shorty," who lived in a small, dilapidated house near the center of Pennington Gap. No one knew where Shorty got her drugs, but it was not through legitimate channels.

In the summer of 1999, Lindsay hung out and got high. She would pick up friends and drive out of Pennington Gap on a narrow country lane called Skaggs Hill Road, which meandered through rugged farm country and onto Skaggs Hill, known as "Pill Hill," before circling back to town. Lindsay and her friends would pull off on one of the road's many turnouts, crush Oxys, and snort them. As the weeks passed, Lindsay and her friends had more and more company. Some days, she saw a different car full of users pulled off along the side of Skaggs Hill Road every quarter mile or so.

It was during the Fourth of July weekend that Lindsay had her first glimpse of the drug's dark side. Her uncle hosted an annual family reunion at his lakefront summer home in Tennessee. Lindsay hadn't brought any Oxys with her, and on her first night away, her legs began to hurt. Even in bed, she couldn't keep them from shaking.

"Mom, my legs are hurting so bad!" Lindsay called out. "Would you rub on them?"

Jane massaged her daughter's legs and soothed her to sleep. But the next night the pain was worse.

Lindsay's cramps weren't cured until she got back to Pennington Gap, drove over to Shorty's house, and bought some Oxys. She awoke the next morning feeling good and a little scared. She hadn't thought she could become addicted to the pills, at least not this easily. Later that day Lindsay told Shorty that she might be hooked.

Jane Myers didn't know anything about Shorty. But by the fall of 1999 she had started to worry about her daughter. Lindsay had trouble getting up in the morning. Her interest in school had fallen off and she had quit the track team. Jane's sister told her she had seen Lindsay hanging out with an older girl who had a reputation for doing drugs. She suggested that Jane find Lindsay a summer job, maybe one at the office of the family's coal business. To Jane, a reserved and attractive woman with red hair, the idea of Lindsay doing drugs was inconceivable. She was a teenager and maybe she was going through some kind of phase, but Jane believed her daughter was at an age where she deserved more independence. Jane thought that Lindsay would talk to her about it if she was having a problem. She didn't want to intrude too much on Lindsay's privacy. Besides, Lindsay seemed to be enjoying cheerleading at football games as much as ever. Jane loved to watch her daughter perform. She would often drive her to away games even if it meant a three-hour trip each way.

One evening in the fall of 1999, Lindsay walked in from a game, threw her bag onto the kitchen table, and went downstairs to join her brother and his friends in the basement. On an impulse, Jane decided to open Lindsay's bag. Inside she found a small tablet and a thin metal tube about an inch long. Jane didn't have a clue what they were.

"Lindsay," she called into the basement, "I want to ask you something."

Lindsay came up and looked nonchalantly at the pill that her mother was holding.

"Oh, I haven't been able to sleep," she told Jane. "Kimberly gave me that to help."

Kimberly, who was Lindsay's cousin, was also at the house that night and, after Lindsay went back to the basement, Jane showed her the pill and asked, "Did you give Lindsay this?"

"I haven't given her anything," Kimberly replied.

Jane felt her stomach drop. She shouted for Lindsay to come upstairs.

"Kim didn't give you this pill," she said. "What is it?"

"It's an Oxy," Lindsay said, with an obstinate, challenging look.

"And what's this?" Jane asked, holding up the short, hollow tube.

"That's what I use to snort it," said Lindsay.

With that, Lindsay stormed off into her room. The next morning Jane called Beth Davies, who ran Pennington Gap's
substance-abuse clinic. Davies said she didn't know much about
OxyContin, but she told Jane that the only way to really know
what was going on was to have Lindsay's urine screened. Jane
balked at the idea. She told Beth that making Lindsay submit to
such a test wasn't fair. If someone found out she had been tested,
rumors would follow. Her school record might be blemished.
She might even be thrown off the cheerleading squad. Jane said
she wouldn't approve a test, but she agreed to bring Lindsay to
Davies's office to talk.

Beth Davies, a small, feisty woman with a gravelly voice and a
shock of short silver hair, was as unlikely a substance-abuse
counselor as one might find. In 1999, she was sixty-six years old,
but she looked a good decade younger and had the energy of
someone half her age. She was also a nun. Sister Beth, as many
people called her, had first come to Appalachia in 1972 after
working in parochial schools in New York and Connecticut as a
teacher and administrator. She decided she wanted to become
more involved in environmental battles and, not long after her
arrival in Lee County, she helped lead the fundraising drive to
build the health clinic in St. Charles, where Art Van Zee worked.

Then in 1979, Davies lost her own long-running battle with
alcoholism. She entered a church-owned treatment facility in
Massachusetts for nuns with substance-abuse problems and decided to change careers. She went to Rutgers University in New
Jersey for training in substance counseling and spent a year in
the roughest neighborhoods of Trenton, New Jersey, working
with alcoholics and heroin addicts.

Since the mid-1980s, Davies and Elizabeth Vines, another

nun who battled alcoholism, had run the Addiction Education Center in an old two-story building in downtown Pennington Gap. Initially, the two women worked almost exclusively with alcoholics. But in the early 1990s, they began to see an increase in the abuse of medications, including tranquilizers and the prescription painkillers. Along with Percocet and Tylox, those drugs included Vicodin and Lortab, two popular prescription painkillers that contained hydrocodone, another narcotic. The medical establishment believed then that hydrocodone posed a lower addiction threat than oxycodone, and federal regulations governing hydrocodone-containing drugs were looser, making them easier for doctors to prescribe. But none of these drugs had prepared Davies and Vines for OxyContin.

Lindsay spent an agonizing weekend waiting for her appointment with Beth Davies. Over those forty-eight hours, Lindsay went through withdrawal, the physical equivalent of shock. When patients or drug abusers use a narcotic, they develop "dependence," a natural process in which the body adapts to the powerful effects of an opioid. Physical dependence is not addiction, but if patients or abusers are suddenly deprived of the drug, they will go into withdrawal. For Lindsay, who had been doing three Oxys a day—one before school, one at lunch, and one before cheerleading practice—the process was excruciating. Her legs ached and jerked far more painfully than they had at her uncle's house. She had flu-like symptoms such as chills, a running nose, and severe headaches. She even suffered periods of delirium. One night that weekend, Lindsay dreamed that she had found an Oxy in her room and snorted it. When she woke up and realized it hadn't happened, she began to cry.

By Monday, Lindsay was looking forward to seeing Beth Davies. Her mother hadn't told her much about the drug counselor, but Lindsay assumed that Beth was young, because her name sounded that way. Lindsay imagined that Beth might become a slightly older friend in whom she could confide.

Jane and Lindsay didn't speak much to each other as they drove downtown in the family Mercedes. But as soon as Lindsay walked into Beth Davies's office and saw her, she shut down. There was no way they would ever connect, she decided. Beth was way too old.

"Can you tell me why you are here?" Davies asked her.

"I haven't done anything," Lindsay said.

"Apparently something is concerning your mother or she wouldn't have called," Davies replied. "What do you think it is?"

"I'm okay," Lindsay said. "She's really making too much of this. She wanted me to come, so that's why I'm here."

Lindsay and Beth didn't forge a connection, but for a month afterward, Lindsay managed to stay clean. Then one afternoon she was cruising around town and saw a friend at a gas station. Lindsay pulled in and the girl gave her a big hug.

"Man, I wish I could find something," Lindsay said.

"You're in luck," her friend replied.

YEARS LATER, no one in Lee County would be able to pinpoint the precise moment in 2000 that OxyContin abuse exploded in their midst. Not physicians like Art Van Zee. Not drug counselors like Beth Davies. Not law-enforcement officials. But as the winter of 2000 slid into spring, Oxys seemed to be everywhere.

Six months earlier, in the fall of 1999, the drug had accounted for just a small fraction of police undercover drug buys in southwestern Virginia. But by the following spring that figure had skyrocketed, in some areas to 90 percent. This flood of pills on the street seemed to have multiple sources. Some unscrupulous doctors were running "pill mills," practices where prescriptions are written without a legitimate purpose in exchange for the price of an office visit. Other doctors were fooled into prescribing the drug to abusers who came in pretending to be patients in pain. People were also forging prescriptions for OxyContin or making duplicate copies of real ones.

Before long, the demand for traditional painkillers like Percocet and Lortab had dried up in Lee County because everyone wanted Oxys. It was as if some exotic new specimen had quietly slipped into the local drug supply and driven out the native species. OxyContin's purity made it easy for recreational users to snort it like cocaine and for serious drug addicts to inject it like heroin.

On the black market, OxyContin had a value of $1 per milligram, meaning that a 20-milligram-strength tablet sold for $20 and a 40-milligram tablet sold for $40. For people like Lindsay Myers, who had thousands of dollars in her bank account, finding the cash to buy Oxys wasn't a problem. Because most people didn't have that kind of money, crime accelerated alongside the abuse of OxyContin. Addicts broke into houses and stole cash and televisions. In some cases, cancer and pain patients awoke to find bottles of OxyContin missing from their medicine cabinets. Forged, stolen, and worthless checks began to paper the region. So many of them were for $40—the street price of a 40-milligram Oxy—that cops would joke upon finding one: "We know where that forty dollars went." People eager to get the drug ran up huge debts on their credit cards, buying things they could quickly convert into cash. Those without credit lines shoplifted items like cigarette lighters or compact discs and sold those. In rural southwestern Virginia, chainsaws were popular targets.

As the drug's abuse intensified, its casualties mounted: During the spring of 2000, each week brought more people into the Addiction Education Center hoping to break their Oxy habits. More overdoses were brought into Lee County Hospital on stretchers. Most of those hospitalized were either teenagers or young adults, some with golf-ball-size abscesses on their arms, a sign they were shooting up the drug with hypodermic needles.

By early April, Vince Stravino, a young physician who worked at the hospital with Art Van Zee, decided that he had seen enough. He called the headquarters of Purdue Pharma in Stamford, Connecticut. His call was routed to a physician on the company's staff.

"We are having bad problems," Stravino said. "We are having withdrawals. This is a horrible problem."

The Purdue doctor said she was surprised to hear that people were abusing the drug and assured Stravino she would look into his complaint. It wasn't until ten months later that the company filed a required report notifying the Food and Drug Administration (FDA) of Stravino's phone call. That filing read in part: "Physician reports that unidentified patients (children, teenagers and adults) using OxyContin (controlled-release oxycodone hydrochloride) for unknown reasons 'come to the hospital with overdoses and abscesses because of injections.' Reportedly, children in the area are 'crushing, snorting and injecting OxyContin.' Additional information is being requested."

Purdue Pharma's report to the FDA also made reference to a follow-up phone call from Stravino that came two months after the first: "Additional information received on 05JUN00 from the reporting physician identifies one patient, a 15-year-old Caucasian male who illegally obtained OxyContin 40 mg. tablets. Reportedly, on '07APR00, the patient took an unknown amount of OxyContin and was found unable to walk, talk coherently at school.' Reportedly, the events ended the same date and the patient had a complete recovery. At the time of this report, the patient is undergoing 'in-patient treatment.' The reporting physician determined that the events were 'definitely' related to OxyContin."

Art Van Zee had a hard time coming to grips with the havoc unfolding around him. Throughout the spring of 2000, he remained focused on the same public-health problems in Lee County that had long been his areas of interest, such as teenage pregnancies and infant nutrition. But his concerns about OxyContin were growing. Van Zee liked research and numbers, so he asked a young medical student to conduct a survey at Lee High that would ask students about their use of tobacco, alcohol, and both legal and illicit drugs. He was stunned when he saw the results—28 percent of the eleventh-graders and 20 percent of the twelfth-graders in Lee High said they had tried OxyContin.

It was then that Van Zee understood something new was happening in his small corner of Appalachia, something beyond the bad things that always happened there—joblessness and problems with alcohol and drugs that seemed to flow from one generation to the next. But he still wondered why it had emerged.

Then, in May, Stravino, a big soccer fan, flew to Boston to see a match. He picked up a copy of *The Boston Globe* and stood transfixed as he read an article in the newspaper about the rampant abuse of a new painkiller in Maine.

The article reported that the drug, OxyContin, was for sale virtually everywhere in rural Washington County, which was located in the state's northern tip. People were traveling hundreds of miles to con prescriptions from doctors by complaining about back pain or migraines. The area had once been a place where people left their doors unlocked, but now crime had surged and drug-treatment centers had been overrun. The situation had reached such a crisis that the United States Attorney in Maine wrote to doctors throughout the state, warning them to be vigilant when prescribing OxyContin.

As soon as Stravino got back to Pennington Gap, he showed the article to Van Zee.

TWO

The War Against Pain

FEW DOCTORS CHANGE HOW MEDICINE IS PRACTICED, BUT Russell K. Portenoy was about to join that select group. By 2000, he had emerged as the superstar of a growing medical movement to use powerful narcotics such as OxyContin to treat chronic pain more aggressively. In his mid-forties, he was already recognized as one of the leading specialists in his area. His reputation as an innovative researcher and thinker had grown so quickly that a major New York City hospital, the Beth Israel Medical Center, had created a pain department expressly to lure him there. Over the previous two decades, Portenoy had written or coauthored more than one hundred scientific articles about pain treatment and contributed to at least twelve books. His confidence and quick, easy wit made him a popular speaker at scientific conferences and medical conventions. These qualities also made him a sought-after consultant for pharmaceutical companies that were producing and marketing pain medications. He appeared on television programs and was frequently quoted in newspaper and magazine articles about pain treatment.

Twenty years earlier, at the beginning of his career, pain treatment as a specialty barely existed. In 1981, when he was a new resident at the Albert Einstein College of Medicine, he was introduced to the hospital's teaching staff, who took turns describing their areas of expertise. After one physician said his focus was pain treatment, Portenoy smiled, thinking the man was joking.

"You can't do pain," replied Portenoy, who has a long face with a neatly trimmed beard. "Pain isn't a disease. It's a symptom."

Two decades later, the demands on his time were so great that patients often waited four months to get an appointment to see him. Those who made it through his doors inhabited a particular circle of hell known as "chronic non-malignant pain," or intense pain from causes other than cancer. Severe, ongoing pain often accompanies cancer, as growing malignant tumors press against sensitive nerves or destroy bone. Recurring episodes of serious pain can also be hallmarks of diseases such as sickle-cell anemia, diabetes, rheumatoid arthritis, and shingles. For many of Portenoy's patients, however, pain thrived as though it had a life of its own, outlasting the injury or illness that had first caused it. This pain often proved resistant to treatment. In these patients, it was as if the nervous system had gone haywire, spewing out a constant stream of signals to the brain that translated as an unrelenting scream of pain.

"Chronic pain" is an umbrella term for conditions that have different causes and symptoms. In some patients, a minor injury like a twisted ankle or the breaking of a tiny wrist bone might cause a leg or an arm to swell, sweat, discolor, and even become palsied. In other patients, severe pain leapt from limb to limb without apparent reason, as though it were playing a game of hide-and-seek. Some patients experienced bolts of "phantom pain" seemingly emanating from a limb long severed from their bodies. Others were rendered nauseous, speechless, or prostrate by migraine headaches, cluster headaches, or trigeminal neuralgia, a condition in which intense, ripping pain sporadically explodes along facial nerves. Still other patients awoke from a surgery or a minor procedure like a cosmetic facelift to find themselves accompanied from that day forward by intense burning pain, as though a doctor's scalpel had nicked a nerve.

Many sufferers are consumed by a single idea: finding relief. One of Portenoy's patients, a school custodian, started experiencing mysterious facial pains. At first he thought the problem would pass, but the episodes continued and the pain, which started on the right side of his face and traveled across it, intensified to the point of being unbearable.

A decade-long medical odyssey began. One doctor gave the man blood-pressure medicine. Another one gave him lithium, a drug prescribed for manic depression. He received migraine treatments and started taking fistfuls of Percocet. His condition continued to worsen, and he was forced to stop working. Eventually, one doctor suggested that he might be able to abort the attacks by breathing in oxygen, so he began to travel everywhere with the type of portable oxygen tank that emphysema sufferers use. When he felt an attack coming on, he would press a thumb against the right side of his face and close one nostril with a finger while breathing in oxygen. It helped, but his misery remained so intense that he considered a dentist's recommendation to have some of his teeth removed. The man's son thought he might be suffering from trigeminal neuralgia, the excruciating facial-pain condition, and brought his father to see a doctor who claimed to have developed a successful surgical approach to the condition. But that doctor told them he couldn't help because he believed the man was suffering from cluster headaches, a syndrome of unknown cause that often affects middle-aged men and produces intense pain episodes. One day, the man's wife saw a television documentary about pain that featured Portenoy. They managed to get an appointment with Portenoy, and his prescription of a strong dose of OxyContin put an end to the man's suffering.

OxyContin didn't work this well for all of Portenoy's patients. But he was a firm believer in the value of long-acting narcotics to treat chronic pain, and he kept similar drugs in his armamentarium. One was fentanyl, the powerful synthetic opioid that was marketed by a unit of Johnson & Johnson in the form of a skin patch under the brand name Duragesic. Another long-acting painkiller was methadone, a substance best known as a maintenance narcotic for heroin addicts, which started its medical life as a pain treatment. Portenoy, like other pain specialists, used different pharmaceuticals to supplement or amplify the effects of narcotics. Several drugs used to control epilepsy, for instance, also worked to effectively dampen pain.

For pain patients, an expert of Portenoy's stature was rarely the first stop. By the time a patient saw him, the person was usually loaded down with years of medical records, X-rays, and diagnostic-test results. For Portenoy and specialists like him, deciphering pain was like trying to solve a puzzle. All of this data provided clues to a patient's condition, but the answer was embedded somewhere within the greater jumble of physical, psychological, social, and emotional conditions of each patient.

"Pain is a little science, a lot of intuition, and a lot of art," Portenoy liked to say.

The most commonplace of medical complaints, pain is also the most subjective, because doctors must rely on patients to describe their pain. Pain can be sharp or dull. It can ache or shoot. It can burn or chill. Some patients describe their pain as mimicking the pounding of a hammer, others as the beating of a drum, and still others as the stabbing of a knife. Each person has a unique pain threshold—the point at which one experiences pain—and people raised in different cultures respond to pain differently. David B. Morris noted in his book *The Culture of Pain* that a study performed in the 1950s at a veterans' hospital in San Francisco found that while Jewish and Italian American patients tended to be uninhibited about expressing pain, patients of Irish or Protestant Anglo-Saxon origin were more tight-lipped.

In rare cases, people are born insensitive to pain. What may seem like an enviable asset is, in fact, a disastrous condition that can cause one to sit calmly on a scalding radiator, oblivious to being severely burned. The most widely cited case involved a Canadian girl referred to in reports as Miss C. In their book, *The Challenge of Pain*, Dr. Ronald Melzack and Dr. Patrick D. Wall wrote that Miss C's congenital insensitivity to pain caused her to bite off the tip of her tongue. As a young woman, she developed severely infected joints because she was able to stand in poses that others would find excruciating. Miss C. succumbed to massive infections when she was twenty-nine.

It was pain's inscrutability that made it an also-ran in the hierarchy of medical specialties. Physicians like problems that they can diagnose and solve, and there is no pain thermometer, pain gauge, or pain meter. A doctor can't send out a patient's blood to find clues about their pain. Technology, be it in the form of an X-ray machine or a more advanced device like an MRI scanner, is sometimes helpful but also notoriously unreliable. While 80 percent of people who complain of back pain have X-rays that show evidence of spinal-disc degeneration, about 70 percent of all adults exhibit disc degeneration on X-rays and have no pain. The science of measuring pain had made such little progress by the end of the twentieth century that one of its key tools was a scale of crude cartoonlike faces ranging from smiling to grimacing.

The history of pain management as a modern medical specialty reaches back only to 1973, less than a decade before
Portenoy began his residency and the year that the International
Association for the Study of Pain was created at a conference in
Seattle, Washington. But physicians, philosophers, priests, and
shamans have studied pain and its causes for millennia, trying
to understand the roles that the body, the mind, and the emo-
tions play in the cause of pain and its sensation. Many ancient
civilizations, such as those in Babylonia, Egypt, and India, believed that pain was experienced in the heart and signaled an
emotional unbalance or an invasion of the body by evil or mis-
chievous spirits. It was a Greek scientist named Galen who, in
the second century B.C., began the first systematic examination
of the nervous system. His work was largely forgotten until the
Renaissance, when physicians realized that the brain constantly
received pain signals, ignoring some and amplifying others. By
the late twentieth century, scientists had unraveled the secrets of
the nervous system even further, discovering specific chemicals
that transmitted pain and others that blocked it.

There also have been relatively few advances in pain treatment. Opium, which comes from the opium poppy, has been
used for thousands of years both to treat pain and to produce
pleasure. Through much of history, doctors believed that opium
was benign, in part because it was the only medicine available to
combat life-threatening conditions like uncontrolled diarrhea.
In his book *Opium: A History,* Martin Booth writes that the drug
was used during the nineteenth century in a host of preparations
like paregoric and laudanum and sold to combat a host of medical ills, including the ill-defined "malaise." Opium was also the
basis of so-called "soothing solutions," potions destitute and
overworked Victorian women gave their babies to quiet them.
These potions were also used on "baby farms," the notorious

orphanages of the same period. The opium drinks rendered infants virtually comatose, damaging some for life.

It was in the early nineteenth century that chemists discovered that much of opium's painkilling power came from a substance that they named morphine, after Morpheus, the Greek god of sleep. Morphine's use in medicine soon became more widespread than opium. Researchers continued to isolate other chemicals from opium, including thebaine, the starting material in the production of oxycodone, the active ingredient in drugs such as Percocet and OxyContin.

It had already become apparent by the mid-nineteenth century that opioids carried a price. By 1900 there were an estimated 300,000 morphine addicts in the United States, including many Civil War veterans, who had gotten addicted to the painkiller while being treated for war-related injuries or illnesses. The condition was so commonplace it was called "soldier's disease." Finally, around World War I, the medical profession recognized morphine's intense, habit-forming potential, and the term "addiction" began to be widely used.

Physicians now viewed narcotic drugs as carrying a high risk of so-called iatrogenic addiction, or addiction induced in a patient in the course of treatment by a doctor. Surveys performed in the 1920s of patients in drug-addiction treatment programs estimated that 9 to 24 percent of addicts had first been given narcotics by a physician while being treated for pain.

By the start of the twentieth century, doctors had another reason to worry. In 1914, the federal government passed the Harrison Act, the nation's first drug law. It was essentially a taxing and record-keeping statute, but five years after it was passed, in 1919, the U.S. Supreme Court issued an opinion that interpreted the Harrison Act as also banning the prescribing of narcotics to those addicted to them. By the late 1930s, more than 25,000 doctors had been charged with offenses related to Harrison Act violations.

Physicians still employed morphine to treat severe pain, particularly the intense suffering experienced by cancer patients. But medical views about morphine's addictive potential, even near the end of a patient's life, affected how the drug was used and resulted in needless agony for cancer patients. As recently as the early 1990s, many doctors prescribed morphine to cancer patients on a so-called PRN basis—medical shorthand for *pro re nata*, or "as needed." Morphine's painkilling effect typically lasted for four hours, so under a PRN-based approach, cancer sufferers were supposed to ask for and receive their next dose of morphine when they felt pain returning. The trouble was that cancer patients didn't immediately get another dose of the drug, even if they begged for it or screamed out in agony. Some doctors and nurses, faced with a patient's desperate demands, heard the prevarications of a suspected drug abuser rather than a cry for help. Because of prevailing medical and social stigmas about narcotics, some medical professionals, as well as some patients, believed that a stiff upper lip was the right approach to pain. Cancer pain treated "as needed" could escalate so sharply that the amount of morphine necessary to subdue it put a patient into a mental stupor.

This horrific situation was the genesis for what became known as the hospice movement. An English physician, Dr. Cicely M. Saunders, was one of its early champions. In 1967 Dr. Saunders opened the first facility, St. Christopher's in London, devoted to the care of those in the final months of life. Her philosophy was that the terminally ill should die a dignified death, not in a sterile hospital but rather in comfortable surroundings, even one's home. She also believed that life's end should be as pain-free as possible.

The hospice movement arrived in the United States in the early 1980s. By then, a few American hospitals—most notably Memorial Sloan Kettering Cancer Center in New York City—had already begun to use morphine more aggressively in cancer care. Experts there believed that a cancer patient should be given morphine routinely, not just when it was asked for, in order to keep the drug's analgesic level constant in the bloodstream and avoid the roller-coaster effect of the PRN approach. The facility's extensive work with morphine demonstrated that, contrary to accepted medical conventions, cancer patients who received large morphine doses didn't become addicted or experience the type of euphoric high that drug abusers do. In time, the work at hospitals like Sloan Kettering changed the way cancer pain was treated throughout the United States.

It also drew attention to what pain experts saw as another, even bigger problem: the inadequate treatment of serious pain unrelated to cancer, or chronic non-malignant pain. These patients—who suffered from conditions as diverse as back pain, arthritis, sickle-cell anemia, and other problems—made up 80 percent of those in constant pain, according to some estimates.

In the mid-1980s, as Russell Portenoy was beginning his career, pain-treatment experts used a variety of methods to treat chronic pain, including surgical procedures, cortisone shots, and alternative approaches such as biofeedback and exercise. There was a furious debate under way about how, or even whether, narcotics should be used.

Many leading pain specialists believed that patients who had chronic pain without a clear origin suffered from a complex mix of physical, psychological, and emotional problems. They were also concerned that a steady regimen of narcotic painkillers for their patients would produce drugged-out zombies, drug abusers, or addicts. There was even evidence that narcotics could intensify, rather than help, some types of pain, by suppressing the body's own pain-fighting system.

Those favoring a non-pharmaceutical approach often saw pain patients as head cases who used complaints about pain as a way to get out of work, emotionally manipulate other people, or obtain drugs. The most common pain complaint—lower-back pain—was rarely diagnosed by doctors prior to World War II. But by 1980, it accounted for an astonishing 5 percent of all doctors' visits. This epidemic of back pain, some specialists believed, had less to do with nerve problems or physical injuries than with work-related stress and job dissatisfaction. Researchers theorized that unhappy employees, after sustaining a relatively minor injury, preferred to drag out their sick leave rather than return to work, and that their depression and susceptibility to pain deepened the longer they remained home. Large financial awards from juries or compensation boards were also thought to play a role. After determining that more than half of a group of pain patients involved in lawsuits had pain rooted in emotional causes rather than physical ones, one researcher dubbed the phenomenon "chronic pain in litigation."

Throughout the 1970s and into the 1980s, many specialists advocated for a multidisciplinary approach to severe pain. Hospital centers based on this method operated at the University of Washington and the University of Miami. Patients entering such programs dropped their painkillers at the door, sometimes by the shopping bag full. Then they were slowly weaned off narcotics to prevent withdrawal and put through a regimen of programs that emphasized physical therapy, psychotherapy, and other techniques, including behavior modification. Patients spent several hours a day doing stretching and strengthening exercises like aerobics and swimming. Since many pain patients suffered from anxiety caused by the anticipation of future attacks, they were taught relaxation and stress-management techniques as substitutes for taking tranquilizers, drugs that were also addicting.

This was the landscape of pain treatment when Russell Portenoy started his residency in 1981. His mentor, Dr. Ronald Kanner, was a pain-treatment activist. He had worked at Memorial Sloan Kettering and believed that many doctors in this country suffered from "opiophobia," a term coined by opioid advocates to describe irrational fears about the addictive powers of these drugs.

In Portenoy, Kanner saw not only an eager acolyte but also a world-class researcher, and he quickly threw him into the fray. Handing him a Bronx telephone book, he told him to call local druggists and ask what Schedule II narcotics—like morphine, Dilaudid, and Percocet—they kept in stock. It turned out that druggists in the Bronx had few narcotic painkillers available, both because opioids were rarely prescribed and because pharmacists feared robberies.

Before long, other doctors were referring pain patients to Portenoy. As he learned about pain in many forms, he observed how difficult it was for patients to get help. One patient, a thirty-five-year-old black man with sickle-cell anemia, told Portenoy that each time he suffered an attack he was forced to go to a hospital and endure hours of pain before a hospital emergency-room doctor would give him just a few painkillers. Portenoy wrote him a prescription for Percocet so he would have a ready supply at home. The man broke down and cried, telling Portenoy that no doctor had ever trusted him before.

Portenoy began a research fellowship at Memorial Sloan Kettering, the cancer center on Manhattan's Upper East Side. The facility had become the nation's first hospital to open a unit specifically devoted to the treatment of patient pain and had appointed as its head a seminal figure in the field, Dr. Kathleen M. Foley. Some physicians might have found Memorial Sloan Kettering—a hospital where many patients made their last, losing stand against cancer—a difficult place to work. Portenoy, who worked as a researcher on Foley's small team, saw it as his job to give comfort. His role, unlike that of an oncologist, wasn't to fight cancer's progress but to make the lives of its sufferers more bearable. "We were the white hats," he said years later. "We didn't feel we had to battle the disease. We didn't feel we would be defeated. You would walk into a room with a person with cancer that has metastasized, and the family is there in despair. But you would walk out of the room having done something to help."

In the mid-1980s, Portenoy and other doctors began to administer a new cancer pain medication, called MS Contin. It was sold by Purdue Frederick, the same company that a decade later would create Purdue Pharma to market OxyContin. MS Contin was a time-release version of morphine, and cancer specialists liked it because it was long-lasting and because it didn't contain additives such as aspirin or acetaminophen, which can cause intestinal bleeding and liver damage.

Portenoy also treated chronic-pain patients without cancer, and in 1986 he published a study coauthored by Kathleen Foley that was entitled "Chronic Use of Opioid Analgesics in Non-Malignant Pain." By research standards, it was a limited study, which involved just thirty-eight Memorial Sloan Kettering patients with a mix of pain conditions such as back or facial pain. But with the imprimatur of the famous cancer hospital, its impact was enormous, and the study would serve as the scientific launching pad for Portenoy's career as well as what became known as the pain-management movement.

The intent behind the study was compassionate. Portenoy ar-

gues in it that there is a "subpopulation" of chronic-pain patients who, having failed to get relief otherwise, might benefit
from the long-term use of powerful narcotics, drugs already
shown to be safe when used in cancer patients. "We conclude
that opioid maintenance therapy can be a safe, salutary, and
more humane alternative to the options of surgery or no treatment in those patients with intractable non-malignant pain and
no history of drug abuse," Portenoy and Foley wrote.

Portenoy soon took to the medical lecture circuit to deliver
that message, giving talks sponsored by either drug companies
or an organization supported by the pharmaceutical industry,
the Dannemiller Foundation. Initially, his advocacy for increased
opioid use wasn't welcome. Experts favoring a multidisciplinary
strategy considered him an "evangelist" for the drug industry.
They argued that while powerful narcotics had subdued his
patients' pain, few of those patients were actually functioning
better.

But a new generation of pain specialists had another view.
Many of them believed that reducing severe and incessant pain
was a laudable goal in itself, and Portenoy, as his reputation
grew, drew large crowds. A pain specialist who attended one of
his lectures said, "When you are the first person bringing a radi-
cal approach, a lot of people want to hear what you have to say."

The 1986 study was only a beginning for Portenoy. Over the
next few years, he authored a series of follow-up reports that
provided both the drug industry and opioid advocates with data
to wield as they pushed for the increased use of narcotic painkillers.

In his papers, Portenoy argued that the high addiction rates
noted by researchers in the 1920s were misleading because they
reflected a skewed population—participants in drug-treatment
programs. Instead, he maintained that when one looked at the

experience of pain patients who had received narcotics in medical settings, the addictive risk of the drugs all but disappeared. There was scant data on the subject. But Portenoy pointed to three reports to support his claim. In the years that followed, these studies and their supposed findings would be cited hundreds of times by opioid advocates and drug companies and adopted by the pain-management movement as a kind of scientific holy trinity.

One of those reports had appeared in 1980 in a major medical journal, *The New England Journal of Medicine*, and reviewed narcotics use and addiction in hospital patients. The second of these studies was published in 1977 in a medical journal, *Headache*, and looked at the use of narcotic painkillers by chronic-headache sufferers. And the third study, which appeared in a 1982 issue of another scientific journal, *Pain*, reviewed the experience of burn patients given narcotics while undergoing an extremely painful procedure called debridement, in which dead skin is removed from living tissue to allow healing.

As characterized by Portenoy, the three reports strongly indicated that patients who hadn't abused drugs before faced little, if any, risk when treated with strong opioids like OxyContin. As he described the hospital study, it had found "only four cases of addiction among 11,882 hospitalized patients," and he reported that the study of chronic-headache sufferers had identified only "three problem cases among 2,369 patients." There was also a similarly low rate of problems, Portenoy said, among pain patients given opioids before undergoing debridement.

Years later Purdue Pharma and its medical allies would point to these same studies and Portenoy's portrayal of them as the basis for the company's claim that powerful narcotics such as OxyContin posed an addiction risk to patients of "less than one percent." But in fact the studies, both individually and collectively, did not contain a shred of scientific evidence about the safety of long-term narcotics use.

The report from *The New England Journal of Medicine*, which was portrayed by Portenoy and others as finding "only four cases of addiction among 11,882 hospitalized patients," wasn't even a study. Instead, the figures were contained in a 1980 letter submitted to the medical publication by two researchers, Dr. Hershel Jick and Dr. Jane Porter, who headed an initiative called the Boston Collaborative Drug Surveillance Program, which was intended to better identify the side effects of dozens of different kinds of prescription medications, not just opioids. Their research also had nothing to do with the safety or risks involved with the long-term use of any drugs, because patients were only monitored while they were in the hospital, not afterward. Dr. Jick would say years later that he and Dr. Porter submitted the statistics about narcotics use to *The New England Journal of Medicine* as a letter because they weren't robust enough to merit a study. He added that one couldn't conclude anything about the risks of long-term narcotics from their study and that neither Dr. Portenoy nor anyone else had contacted him before using his research to make misleading claims about it.

Portenoy and others also mischaracterized the study about migraine sufferers. That research had taken place in Chicago at a facility called the Diamond Headache Clinic and looked at the experience of 2,369 patients treated there. But while Portenoy and others claimed that the study had found only "three problem cases" among that large group, that wasn't even close to the facts. Instead, those three problem cases had occurred within a much smaller group of patients, sixty-two of whom were looked at separately because they had taken either painkillers or a combination of painkillers and barbiturates for at least six months before coming to the clinic. Those three patients represented

5 percent of that group, and Portenoy, even while touting the headache report, had neglected to cite its conclusion. The study specifically warned against the use of narcotics in headache sufferers, stating: "There is a danger of dependency and abuse in patients with chronic headaches."

Years later, long after OxyContin had cut its swath of destruction through places like Lee County, Portenoy would issue a cautious apology about his failure to properly cite the studies. He said that he had wanted to create a "narrative" that would diminish negative attitudes about opioids and help pain patients receive better care. But during his days as the champion of the pain-management movement, his assertion of the safety of long-term opioid use was often unequivocal and unvarnished. "There is a growing literature showing that these drugs can be used for a long time, with few side effects, and that addiction and abuse are not a problem," he told one newspaper reporter.

There is little question that when Portenoy promoted his opioid narrative in the early 1990s, the medical profession needed to change how pain was treated. Many physicians received only an hour of training in medical school about pain and its management. Doctors, concerned about the possibility of addiction, also resisted prescribing strong opioids. A 1991 survey of state medical-board members conducted by researchers at the University of Wisconsin reported that only 12 percent of board members viewed such treatment as acceptable practice. The way of treating severe pain in some groups of patients—in particular, the elderly and newborns—bordered on the barbaric. Up until the mid-1980s, surgeons operated on desperately ill newborns without using painkillers, because they were considered too risky for infants to tolerate. For years, children in pain were inadequately medicated. "Most adults would be shocked if they saw what was done to children in hospitals without anesthetics," one pediatric-pain expert told the *Los Angeles Times* in 1991.

Spurred by leaders of the pain-management movement, government authorities soon began calling for better care. In 1992, for example, a unit of the Public Health Service called the Agency for Health Care Policy issued new guidelines that urged hospitals to use powerful narcotics more aggressively to treat the type of acute pain experienced as the result of surgery. Dr. James O. Mason, the Public Health Service's top official, said the new recommendations were needed to dispel "cultural" myths that pain "is necessary to build character, that infants do not feel pain, that elderly patients have a higher pain tolerance, and that narcotics used for postoperative pain are often addictive."

Opioid advocates also had begun to make slow but steady progress on another critical front: convincing state legislators or state medical boards—the agencies in each state that license doctors—to encourage a more liberal use of strong painkillers. Beginning with Texas in 1989, a growing number of states passed laws or adopted medical guidelines that specifically recognized the value of powerful narcotics in treating severe chronic pain. Opioid advocates had long argued that new rules were necessary because narcotics agents and medical regulators had unfairly targeted doctors who used large amounts of painkillers.

All advocacy movements need good bogeymen, and pain-management activists had long identified their enemy as any law, any institution, or any regulatory mechanism that deterred doctors from liberally prescribing opioids. Among those roadblocks, they argued, were databases used by some states to track a physician's dispensing of controlled substances, or "prescription-monitoring systems," as they are known.

In the mid-1990s, such systems existed in only fourteen states, and law-enforcement authorities used them to identify doctors who wrote an unusually high volume of prescriptions for opioids. In some cases, those numbers might simply reflect the nature of a doctor's specialty. But in other cases, a large number of prescriptions for painkillers could be a sign that a physician was running a "pill mill." States such as New York, which monitored prescriptions for Schedule II narcotics like morphine and oxycodone, had typically adopted the systems in response to outbreaks of prescription-drug abuse.

For years, both drug companies and the American Medical Association, the professional group that represents doctors, had fiercely opposed prescription monitoring. But as the pain-management movement gathered strength in the early 1990s, opioid advocates took over a leading role in that campaign, arguing that prescription monitoring was having a "chilling effect" on legitimate prescribing, because doctors feared landing on law enforcement's radar.

A leading voice opposing monitoring was the head of a think tank at the University of Wisconsin, David E. Joranson. Originally called the Pain Treatment Group, the research organization later changed its name to the Pain and Policies Studies Group. Earlier in his career, Joranson had been the administrator of Wisconsin's Controlled Substances Board, where he became involved in the late 1980s in efforts to improve cancer-pain care in the state. Soon afterward, he left government and devoted himself to pain-care advocacy, including promoting better cancer-pain treatment in developing countries, where taboos against morphine still existed.

But in a series of papers in the early 1990s, Joranson argued that prescription monitoring was of little proven law-enforcement value and that it was causing doctors to limit writing narcotics prescriptions for patients who needed the drugs. Publicly, Joranson stated he favored an approach to monitoring that "balanced" the needs of law enforcement and pain patients. But for opioid activists, "balance" became a word used to mask an agenda. For example, when several states tried to accommodate complaints from physicians about prescription monitoring by switching from paper forms to electronic ones, Joranson opposed that too. "Requiring the use of these prescription forms would send an unmistakable message to physicians that prescribing controlled substances could give them an unwanted high profile with the police or licensing authorities if they order more than a minimal amount for patients in pain," Joranson and a coauthor wrote in a 1993 issue of a pro-opioid publication, the *American Pain Society Bulletin*.

At the time some medical experts, such as Dr. Sidney Wolfe of the Health Research Group, an advocacy group critical of the drug industry, argued that there was little evidence to support the claim by Joranson and others that prescription monitoring had a "chilling effect" on medical practice. But by the mid-1990s, the pain-management movement was strong enough to defeat a congressional initiative to create a prescription-monitoring system at both the state and national levels.

By then the news media was also carrying the movement's message to the public. Within the space of two months during the spring of 1997, *U.S. News & World Report* published an article entitled "The Quality of Mercy," while *Forbes* published "The Morphine Myth." Some journalists trumpeted the data from the three studies that Portenoy cited as showing that narcotics held scant addiction risk for patients, without ever looking to see what the studies really said.

Other writers chose to dramatize the battle against pain, describing how medical "myths," intrusive regulations, or meddling government drug agents were depriving patients of desperately needed medications. In 1997, *Playboy* magazine even suggested that the U.S. government, "needing a winnable war . . . had cracked down on doctors' offices." The article continued:

> Across the country, state agents, allied with the DEA, have staked out pain clinics under the assumption that wherever narcotics are prescribed, diversion of the drugs will soon follow. In pursuing this theory, the government has criminalized an entire class of patients and scared doctors into abandoning them.

Journalists were missing important stories, however, about the misuse of science and the network of financial ties between the pain-management movement and the drug industry. Industry money supported not only research by investigators such as Russell Portenoy but also the work of consultants and virtually every pain-management specialist advocating for increased opioid prescriptions. Drug companies also spent heavily to subsidize "patient" advocacy groups such as the American Pain Foundation and the two principal professional groups representing pain specialists, the American Pain Society (APS) and the American Academy of Pain Medicine (AAPM). In 1997 alone, Purdue Pharma contributed half a million dollars to underwrite the work of a joint committee formed by the two groups, which issued a report urging the broader medical application of powerful narcotics.

Drug companies also funded David Joranson's Pain and Policies Studies Group at the University of Wisconsin. While the group did receive support from some nonprofit organizations, such as the Robert Wood Johnson Foundation, the majority of its funding came from such makers of opioids as Janssen Pharmaceuticals, Knoll Pharmaceuticals, and Ortho-McNeil. The most generous of these industry donors was Purdue, which gave Joranson's group hundreds of thousands of dollars.

Ideological ties between opioid advocates and a company like Purdue were even more powerful than financial ones. Many experts calling for a more aggressive use of narcotics viewed Purdue not as a profit-seeking enterprise but as an ally in a noble social cause—the betterment of pain treatment. "I view them as our colleagues in education," Kathleen Foley, Russell Portenoy's colleague at Memorial Sloan Kettering, said in a 1996 interview. "It was not the government that wanted to educate; it was not the National Cancer Institute that wanted to educate. It was the drug company that wanted to improve pain management." Pain experts would find these ties hard to shake when OxyContin abuse exploded.

Many doctors watched with dismay as the agendas of professional groups like the American Pain Society shifted to reflect a pharmacological approach to treatment. "The APS should really stand for the American Pharmaceutical Society," said one clinical psychologist. The influence of those championing non-drug approaches to chronic pain was fading for other reasons as well. Studies indicated that chronic-pain patients who entered multidisciplinary programs at places like the University of Miami emerged improved but had high relapse rates. The era of managed care was also in full throttle, and those who treated pain faced the same economic pressures as psychotherapists. Insurers were willing to pay for pills but not for the therapy and rehab regimes at multidisciplinary centers, which could cost up to $20,000.

A few voices of dissent were raised. In a 1996 paper published in the *Journal of Pain and Symptom Management*, one pain specialist, Dr. Dennis Turk, argued that the views of the opposing experts—the advocates for a multidisciplinary approach to pain management and those favoring opioids—were both mistaken, because their perspectives had been molded by small, unique groups of patients. Turk maintained that multidisciplinary disciples unfairly dismissed narcotics because drugs hadn't worked for patients who presented extremely difficult cases. He cautioned that opioid champions were projecting their experience based on an equally limited group—cancer patients—across the wide realm of pain sufferers.

In that same publication, a leading authority on substance abuse, Dr. Seddon R. Savage of Dartmouth Medical School, sounded a different warning. Savage argued that the typical rate of substance abuse found in the general population—a range of 3 to 16 percent, with 10 percent the most referenced figure—might also hold true for pain patients put on strong narcotics for long periods. She also noted that the risk of addiction in pain patients was likely to rise the longer they used opioids. "It is tempting to dismiss all concerns regarding therapeutic opioids use as irrelevant," Savage wrote in 1996, adding:

> That would clearly be a mistake. Many pain specialists who enthusiastically embraced the possibility of long-term opioid therapy for the treatment of chronic pain have been startled by the unanticipated consequences of such use, which were not observed in previous experience with acute pain and cancer pain because the clinical variables in each of these settings differ significantly. Historical cautions regarding opioids use are not without basis.

Around 1990, Russell Portenoy made a trip to the headquarters of Purdue, then located in Norwalk, Connecticut. He met with top company executives and scientists and urged them to develop a strong, long-acting opioid that doctors could give to chronic-pain patients. Portenoy would later recall that company officials did not appear enthusiastic about his idea. He said he suspected that the reason was simple: At the time, both doctors and patients thought of long-acting opioids such as Purdue's MS Contin as drugs of last resort that carried the stigma of terminal illness.

"I never heard back from them," Portenoy said. "I just assumed that it was too hot, the connotation was too negative."

By the time of Portenoy's visit, however, the idea for that drug, which would be called OxyContin, was already on Purdue's drawing board, and the company would soon launch a massive campaign to change how doctors thought about narcotics. Portenoy had laid groundwork for this campaign, but the little-known family that owned Purdue, the Sacklers, brought something indispensable to the effort—a mastery of pharmaceutical marketing.

Years later, a sales rep hired by Purdue to promote OxyContin recalled the initial meeting with one of the three Sackler brothers who had helped start Purdue, Dr. Raymond Sackler. He was already eighty, but he tried to meet with new hires. Raymond Sackler waxed enthusiastic during the rep's visit to his office about the prospects for OxyContin and how it would turn Purdue into a pharmaceutical powerhouse. "OxyContin," he declared, "is our ticket to the moon."

THREE

Secrets of Dendur

FOUR DECADES BEFORE RAYMOND SACKLER PINNED HIS hopes on OxyContin, his oldest brother, Dr. Arthur M. Sackler, sat before a panel of U.S. senators. They had called him to testify during a 1962 hearing investigating the promotion of pharmaceuticals with misleading claims or tactics.

Today, drug companies advertise and market prescription medications directly to doctors as a matter of course. But in 1962 the pharmaceutical industry had only recently adopted this strategy, and critics were concerned that it would lead to deceptive promotions and corrupt medicine. Arthur Sackler headed the country's largest advertising agency devoted to the marketing of pharmaceuticals, William Douglas McAdams in New York City. That agency was only the most visible symbol of Sackler's dominance of the promotional end of the drug industry. His web of business interests was so vast and complex that details about its full extent would emerge only after his death.

Arthur Sackler was a complex person of extraordinary will and determination, lionized by his friends and admirers as a Renaissance man with a passion for science and an entrepreneurial vision that allowed him to pursue multiple careers simulta-

neously. Even while he was a medical student, he was employed
as a drug-advertising copywriter. He later served as the head of a
major psychiatric research institute while working as a pharmaceutical marketing executive.

Starting in the 1940s, Sackler created a sprawling drug industry, encompassing every aspect of the way drugs were made,
marketed, advertised, and sold. While his advertising agency
created promotional campaigns for prescription drugs, Sackler
consulted with some of the world's biggest drug companies,
helping them define the medical conditions for which their medications would be marketed as cures. He also controlled a chain
of scientific journals that carried research articles about new
drugs and provided favorable reports about those produced by
his advertising clients. A biweekly newspaper he owned, the
Medical Tribune, was distributed free to 168,000 doctors nationwide, and its views often echoed those of the drugmakers that
advertised in it.

Sackler also created less obvious, though no less effective,
outlets for his clients to reach doctors and the ultimate consum-
ers of drugs, patients. Sackler presided over the birth of the in-
fomercial, a means of pharmaceutical promotion that would
become ubiquitous. In the 1960s, various firms he controlled
created and distributed free "articles" to newspapers and other
publications that were really marketing plugs for products sold
by his drug-company clients. Purdue would later use this strategy in an effort to boost OxyContin sales, distributing "surveys"
to spotlight the inadequate treatment of pain.

In his 1962 Senate appearance, Arthur Sackler faced hostile
questioning from a formidable adversary, the legendary senator
Estes Kefauver, the Tennessee Democrat. That same year, Kefauver had sounded one of the first public alarms about thalido-
mide, a tranquilizer that caused birth defects, and he was a

leading critic of how the pharmaceutical industry tested and marketed drugs. While questioning Sackler, Kefauver asked him about his ties to a small public-relations company called Medical and Science Communications Associates, a firm that distributed promotional news articles.

Sackler acknowledged to the senators that William Douglas McAdams worked with Medical and Science Communications. But he adamantly denied that he had any influence over the public-relations firm's activities, even though it happened to be located at the same Lexington Avenue address in New York as his ad agency.

"I never had any stock in Medical and Science Communications, and I was never an officer," Sackler avowed.

Strictly speaking, his sworn testimony was accurate. The corporate paperwork for Medical and Science Communications did not list him as either a company officer or a shareholder. But in fact the company's sole shareholder was Else Sackler, Arthur's ex-wife and the first of three women he would marry. It was common practice for Arthur Sackler to put the names of his wives, children, or business associates on corporate documents to shield his own involvement.

Sackler walked away unscathed from the Senate hearing, his reputation unblemished. He had handled himself confidently, referring frequently to his extensive medical credentials—his directorship of a research facility, his publication of sixty scientific papers, his memberships in prestigious organizations—as proof that the advertisements created by his agency were based on science, not hyperbole. While quietly displaying his contempt for bureaucrats and lawmakers, he had managed to keep the details of his business dealings private. Like the marketing genius he was, Arthur Sackler had created an illusion and then disappeared.

All three Sackler brothers, who founded Purdue, preferred to operate in secrecy, but this was especially true of Arthur, the undisputed head of the family. He lived by one guiding star and played by one set of rules—his own. Whatever the names on corporate documents or letterheads, Arthur controlled everything in his realm, even at times his brothers, Mortimer and Raymond.

"In my mind, it was all Arthur," a top executive at William Douglas McAdams told a lawyer after Sackler's death, to explain the business ties between him and his brothers. "I guess legally you had to break it out into different, quote, 'affiliated' companies, and these are the legal entities. But, actually, to me the whole thing was Arthur."

Sackler spent the last years of his life using the massive fortune he had earned to acquire world-renowned collections of Asian antiquities, European bronzes, and exquisite majolica ceramics. He counted Linus Pauling, the Nobel Prize–winning chemist, among his friends. He talked art and politics with Anwar Sadat, the president of Egypt, and Moshe Dayan, the Israeli defense minister. He socialized with some of the cultural icons of his day, such as the painter Marc Chagall, the sculptor Isamu Noguchi, and the opera singer Richard Tucker.

Today, the Sackler name adorns museums, medical schools, and other institutions worldwide. Along with his younger brothers, Arthur Sackler financed the construction of the Sackler Wing at the Metropolitan Museum of Art in New York City. A striking glass-curtained addition, it houses treasures from the age of the Egyptian pharaohs, most notably the Temple of Dendur, a large stone shrine supported by two columns that was transported to New York and rebuilt inside the Sackler Wing. There is the Arthur M. Sackler Gallery at the Smithsonian Institution in Washington, D.C., the Arthur M. Sackler Museum at Harvard University in Massachusetts, and the Arthur M. Sackler Museum of Art and Archaeology at Peking University in China.

His giving gained Sackler entry to a tier of society far above his humble origins. The son of Jewish immigrants from Eastern Europe, he was born and grew up in the Flatbush section of Brooklyn, New York, then a working-class neighborhood. His father's business failed during the Depression, and he later opened a small grocery store. To help his family financially, Arthur sold ads for local newspapers and other publications. He graduated from New York University in 1933 and went on to get his medical degree from the same school.

From the beginning, he comfortably juggled different careers. In 1944, he became both president of William Douglas McAdams and a psychiatric resident at Creedmoor State Hospital in Queens, New York. Even as his advertising business flourished, Arthur rose through the ranks at Creedmoor, a hospital for the mentally ill, and eventually became director of a research center there called the Institute for Psychobiologic Studies. By the 1950s, Sackler was already wealthy enough from his drug-advertising business to subsidize the institute where he worked. If not for the financial lures of a business career, Arthur Sackler might have gone on to be a prominent research scientist. He played a role in early efforts to understand the chemistry of mental illness. In the early 1950s, he and associates at Creedmoor published numerous papers that suggested the blood chemistry of schizophrenics was different from that of emotionally healthy people. They attempted to develop blood tests to screen for serious mental illness as well.

Sackler was also the godfather of the modern-day drug-advertising industry, inventing or refining many of the marketing and promotional techniques still used decades later by pharmaceutical producers. At one time, drug companies didn't directly advertise prescription drugs to doctors, and certainly not in medical publications. But Arthur Sackler changed all that, transforming both the pharmaceutical industry and the practice of medicine in the process.

After World War II, when Sackler's advertising career took off, the pharmaceutical industry was going through a transformation. Drugmakers started to greatly expand the types of medications they produced while shortening the life span of each drug they manufactured in order to make way for "new" or "improved" versions. It was the era of the "wonder" drug, as waves of new antibiotics, tranquilizers, psychotropic drugs, and other medications appeared, each offering the hope that it could cure a previously untreatable illness.

Historically, drug-company sales reps were the ones who introduced physicians to a new medication. But in 1952, Arthur Sackler engineered the insertion of a multipage color advertisement in the *Journal of the American Medical Association* (*JAMA*), one of the nation's leading medical journals, promoting a new antibiotic sold by Pfizer Laboratories. It was the first time a drug advertisement had appeared in a major journal, and it heralded an era of increasing financial entanglements between drug companies and doctors.

Arthur Sackler believed that the advertising, marketing, and promotion of drugs played a vital role in keeping physicians aware of the rapidly changing landscape of medications available to them. In a 1950s interview, he remarked that only about 20 percent of the money pharmaceutical makers directed toward drug advertising was spent on direct brand promotion. Instead, the vast bulk of such funds, he explained, was used for the education of physicians.

"The bulk of money being spent [on advertising] is primarily for informational and educational uses," he was quoted as saying. "The term 'advertising budget' is therefore a misnomer. This 'promotion' is as essential for the safe and proper use of drugs as good driving and accident-prevention campaigns are for the safe and proper use of automobiles."

Under the rubric of physician education, Sackler breathed life into another way to market drugs. Inspired by Sackler's example, virtually every pharmaceutical company had begun to sponsor so-called continuing-medical-education courses for health professionals, or CMEs. These were hour-long talks about medical issues that also served as vehicles to pitch or promote new pharmaceuticals. Decades later, Purdue would spend a small fortune underwriting CMEs about the inadequate treatment of pain and the need for doctors to address it more aggressively by using long-acting narcotics like OxyContin.

Arthur Sackler not only created new ways to market drugs, he helped create a new chapter in American life—the emergence of the pill as a quick fix. The feel-good tranquilizers of the 1960s, Librium and Valium, were immortalized in Jacqueline Susann's novel *Valley of the Dolls* and the Rolling Stones' hit song "Mother's Little Helper." It was Arthur Sackler's marketing genius that turned Librium and Valium into staples in medicine chests and nightstands throughout the United States, two of the greatest promotional successes of their era.

Pharmacologically, Librium and Valium belonged to the same class of drugs, known as benzodiazepines. Both drugs worked similarly to calm a patient's nerves and were also potentially addicting. But Arthur, working as a consultant to the drugs' producer, Hoffmann–La Roche of Switzerland, skillfully promoted them as though they were two entirely different medications.

Doctors could then prescribe them for different problems and the two products would not cannibalize each other's sales. He positioned Librium, which was launched first, as a treatment for "anxiety" while promoting Valium for a separate set of mental concerns and preoccupations that he called "psychic tension."

Using that battle plan, Roche Labs, Hoffmann–La Roche's subsidiary in the States, promoted its twin tranquilizers, spending between $150 million and $200 million, numbers unheard of in the pharmaceutical industry. As John Pekkanen described it in his 1973 book, *The American Connection*, the money was used to unleash an unprecedented marketing campaign for Librium and Valium, aimed at both doctors and the public. Pekkanen wrote:

> The whole drug industry campaign for mood drugs in the 1960s was to broaden to absurd limits the definition of illness to include every upset, every disappointment, and every vague problem encountered in day-to-day living. Each was a ripe candidate for drug-taking. If the facts in these ads were not untruths, then their implications often were. Roche Labs pushed its tranquilizer twins for a variety of "illnesses," although they were careful never to urge the use of Librium and Valium for treatment of the same problem. But the cumulative effect of the advertising in medical journals was to cover every problem encountered in a doctor's office: tension, anxiety, muscle spasms, even something called the "intervals," described as that worrisome time when one wonders about some dark possibility in the future. Rapid pulse, faintness, breathlessness, missed periods, hot flashes, fear, and depression were all apt candidates

for either tranquilizers, stimulants, depressants, or antidepressants, or all of those. There was a chemical solution for everything.

Arthur Sackler, already a rich man, made an emperor's fortune from Librium and Valium. Under the terms of his agreement with Hoffmann–La Roche, he received bonus payments
based on the volume of pills sold. The Swiss drugmaker, grateful
to Sackler for the drugs' success, provided him with millions of
dollars in interest-free loans as advances against future advertising work, money that he quickly invested to make yet another
fortune in the stock market.

While many saw Arthur Sackler's career as the rise of a self-
made man, others viewed him as a relentless and sometimes
ruthless competitor who hid his pursuit of profit behind a veil of
science. In transforming the drug-advertising industry, he also
helped pioneer some of its most controversial and troubling
practices: the showering of favors on doctors, the lavish spending on consultants and experts ready to back a drugmaker's
claims, the funding of supposedly independent medical interest
groups, the creation of publications to serve as industry mouth-
pieces, and the outright expropriation of scientific research for
marketing purposes.

His advertising firms used promotional gimmicks that seemed
more like the work of a huckster plying the frontiers of a wild
and untamed industry than the product of legitimate science.
Sackler's firm produced a brochure for Pfizer Laboratories promoting an antibiotic called Sigmamycin that depicted the supposed business cards of several physicians in various cities as
though they were testimonials to the drug's effectiveness. The
cards showed each physician's address, telephone number, and

office hours. But when a curious journalist tried to contact doctors cited in the ad, he found they didn't exist.

Copywriters working for Arthur Sackler also reshaped the work of real doctors and medical researchers. In the 1950s, an ad announcing the discovery of a "happy baby vitamin" appeared in a free weekly newsletter produced by William Douglas McAdams and distributed to doctors on behalf of the Upjohn Company, a major drugmaker. That vitamin—pyridoxine, or B6—also happened to be an ingredient in an Upjohn product called Zymabasic Drops. The advertisement, which depicted a sleep-deprived father holding an infant, read:

> The wakeful baby who turns father into a floor walker may simply lack B6. Infant's formula and mother's milk frequently fail to provide sufficient amounts of this "happy baby vitamin." That's why basic baby supplementation calls for Zymabasic, the formula with all four: A, D, and C, plus B6.

In 1958, Dr. Charles B. May, the editor of *Pediatrics*, the medical journal of the American Academy of Pediatrics, decided to investigate. Alarmed by the sudden bevy of infant supplements containing B6, he contacted several scientists to determine whether Upjohn and other drugmakers were advertising their research properly.

"I would appreciate your letting me know if you believe your work had been properly exploited by those who urge its universal use as a supplement to the infant's diet," May wrote in July 1958 to those researchers. Their reaction was a uniform "no." One of them, Arild E. Hansen of the University of Texas, replied that his work on the effect of B6 on colicky babies was so pre-

liminary and inconclusive that he had dropped it. "Never by any
stretch of the imagination have we inferred that there is such a
thing as a 'happy baby vitamin,'" Dr. Hansen wrote. He and the
other scientists all said that no one from Arthur Sackler's firm or
Upjohn had informed them that their research was being cited
in product promotions. More than four decades later, Dr. Hershel Jick of the Boston Collaborative Drug Surveillance Program
would find himself in much the same situation, with OxyContin.

As the lord of his realm, Arthur Sackler didn't hesitate to make
careers or crush them, inspiring both loyalty and terror among
his employees and business associates. He used his vast empire
of publications to promote the interests of his friends and corporate allies and to savage others. One favored vehicle for his personal philosophies and political views was the *Medical Tribune*,
the newspaper Sackler distributed to doctors. In the *Tribune*, he
wrote a column called "One Man and Medicine," which dispar-
aged regulators as overreaching, sang the praises of unbridled
scientific research, and occasionally took potshots at other in-
dustries. He hated cigarettes and lambasted automakers for fail-
ing to quickly install seatbelts. He also used the *Medical Tribune*
to protect his drug-industry clients, particularly the big pharmaceutical companies that produced brand-name prescription
medications.

Apart from government regulators, Sackler and his clients
had no greater enemy than manufacturers of "generic" drugs,
companies that waited until a name-brand drug's patent expired
and then made a cheaper version of it. Sackler contended that
generic drugs were not necessarily as effective as their more expensive rivals, and his *Medical Tribune* published articles about
generics depicting them as the pharmaceutical equivalent of a
Red menace. One of these, entitled "Schizophrenics 'Wild' on
Weak Generic," described how "all hell broke loose" at a Veter-

ans Administration hospital after patients were switched from the brand-name antipsychotic drug Thorazine to a generic equivalent. The article went on to relate that eleven previously stabilized patients had run amok until they were switched back to Thorazine, at which point their behavior returned to normal "as if a switch had been flipped." FDA officials investigated the episode and found that the report cited in the *Medical Tribune* was so scientifically flawed as to be useless in determining the safety of the generic.

Arthur's two brothers, Mortimer and Raymond, were highly intelligent and accomplished men who would also go on to give generously to the arts, science, and medicine. But they were a part of Arthur's world and spent much of their lives working in his shadow. Arthur was three years older than Mortimer and seven years older than Raymond, but he treated them more like progeny and understudies than siblings. He got them into medical schools, paid for their training as research psychiatrists, and arranged jobs for them at the Creedmoor research facility he funded. Dr. Stanley Graham, a psychiatrist in New York who worked at the institute in the early 1950s, later recalled that Arthur treated his brothers like hired help. "He told everyone exactly what to do, including Morty and Ray," Graham remembered.

When Mortimer and Raymond were fired from Creedmoor in 1953, after refusing to sign a McCarthy-era loyalty oath, Arthur stepped in and found his brothers new work. He set them up in the business of making drugs.

FOR YEARS, Arthur Sackler had watched his pharmaceutical-advertising clients grow rich manufacturing products for pennies and selling them at huge markups. Sackler wanted a piece of this business, but he couldn't compete with his advertising clients, so he did the next best thing. He financed the purchase of a drug company and let his brothers run it.

It was called the Purdue Frederick Company. Located on Christopher Street in New York's Greenwich Village, it had roots stretching back to 1892, an era of feel-good elixirs and patent medicines that owed their revitalizing or curative powers to opiates, alcohol, or a combination of the two. Founded by Dr. John Purdue Gray and George Frederick Bingham, Purdue Frederick made a cure-all called Gray's Glycerine Tonic Compound, which contained a generous serving of sherry and was one of the company's biggest sellers for several decades. An advertising card sent to physicians in 1937 read: "When Spring Comes Gray's Glycerine Tonic Comp. should be a suggestion to your patient— tired from Winter Ills. Prescribe this dependable Tonic which has stood 'The Test of Time' for over forty-five (45) years." When the Sacklers acquired the company in 1952, it had annual revenues of only $22,000.

Purdue's first products under Sackler-family management did not suggest it would one day produce powerful painkillers like OxyContin. In 1955, Purdue started selling a brand of laxatives under the name Senokot and three years later added the prescription earwax remover Cerumenex to its product line. (Both were successful and are still sold by the company.) On the basis of his experience in the pharmaceutical industry, Arthur Sackler, who likely had a role in acquiring Senokot and Cerumenex, knew that a small, privately held operation such as Purdue would prosper only if it found opportunities or created niches unclaimed by big manufacturers. Decades later, this idea led his brothers to see opportunity in another overlooked area—the treatment of pain.

In the 1950s, Purdue Frederick was only one of several drug-related businesses run by Mortimer and Raymond Sackler.

They also owned the Glutavite Corporation, which sold a product called l-Glutavite. *Medical Tribune* advertisements depicted aging men and women and described l-Glutavite as a "metabolic cerebral tonic" capable of revitalizing confused minds. Despite its quasi-medical name, l-Glutavite was a throwback to the era of patent medicines. It was nothing more than a mixture of monosodium glutamate—the meat tenderizer known as MSG—and vitamin B. The ads promoting it as a mental stimulant were the handicraft of the drug industry's dream factory, Arthur Sackler's William Douglas McAdams agency.

The explosive growth of the drug-marketing industry in the late 1950s caught the attention of the science editor of the influential *Saturday Review*, John Lear. He saw the promotional onslaught as a threat to public health. Producers encouraged the use of different antibiotics at the same time to treat a patient, a dangerous practice that can create drug-resistant bacteria. Lear began a series of investigative articles that sought to undo the growing interdependence of a drug's production and its promotion.

Decades earlier, Lear had made his reputation by exposing a scam in the Agriculture Department. Now his reporting trail led him straight toward the three Sackler brothers and the government agency entrusted with regulating the drug industry, the FDA.

The initial target of Lear's investigation was an FDA official named Henry Welch, who was in charge of the division that regulated antibiotics. Lear discovered that Welch was on the payroll of two journals that published research reports about those drugs, *Antibiotics and Chemotherapy* and *Antibiotic Medicine and Clinical Therapy*. When Lear confronted him about his payments from the publications, Welch insisted that his ties did not pose a conflict of interest, because the journals were indepen-

dent of the pharmaceutical industry. A congressional investigation prompted by a Lear article found, however, that the $287,000
the publications paid to Welch over a six-year period came from
the very antibiotic producers he regulated. The drug manufacturers had spent millions buying reprints of articles that appeared in the journals and distributed them as sales tools to
doctors. Welch's payout reflected his cut of the take, a 7½ percent royalty from reprint sales. Not incidentally, drugmakers got
to read and edit research articles about their antibiotics before
they appeared in print.

Welch immediately resigned in disgrace. Lear continued dig-
ging and discovered that drug companies paid a company called
MD Publications for the reprints they bought, and it paid Welch
his share. The president of MD Publications was a researcher
named Dr. Felix Marti-Ibanez, but Lear suspected he was just a
figurehead used to shield the company's true owners.

Marti-Ibanez was also an employee of a branch of Arthur
Sackler's advertising agency, and MD Publications shared its office space. He had also worked alongside Arthur Sackler and his
two brothers at Creedmoor. Welch had acknowledged to Lear
that Marti-Ibanez shared the ownership of MD Publications
with two other investors but didn't reveal their identities. Lear
thought he had a pretty good idea that they were two of the three
Sackler brothers.

In a March 1962 article of *The Saturday Review,* Lear introduced readers to them. He depicted the Sacklers as modern-day
moguls whose influence over the new industry of drug promotion was akin to John D. Rockefeller's dominance of the oil industry or Jay Gould's seizure of the railroads. He described the
Sackler brothers' production, promotion, and advertising of
l-Glutavite as emblematic of the far greater change taking place

throughout the pharmaceutical industry—its evolution into a mass-marketing machine for pills.

> The spectacle of three psychiatrists, members of a profession looked to with almost awesome respect for guidance in mental illness, concertedly pushing a flavoring extract mixed with vitamins as a means of arresting the pitiable deterioration of aging minds, is a painful experience. But the l-Glutavite episode has significance beyond the compass of psychiatry. It illustrates the machine-like disregard of individuality in which the once precise art of prescription drug administration has descended in America.
>
> The combined resources of the three Sackler brothers for this type of integrated drug marketing were not exhausted in the promotion of l-Glutavite. The brothers cover every aspect of prescription medicine. They have succeeded in carrying out their operation despite opposition within the medical profession. Whatever opposition they may have encountered within the drug industry itself has not been effective.

Then he made his case for the connection between Henry Welch, MD Publications, and the Sacklers. He tried to piece together a tangled business trail, one made more impenetrable because the companies involved were private and so didn't have to disclose their true ownership. Names involved with the Sacklers kept popping up, including that of a lawyer and an accountant who had done work for Arthur. Lear noted that a news agency owned by Arthur was the first to announce in 1951 that Welch would edit a new journal called *Antibiotics and Chemistry*.

He also discovered that Mortimer Sackler sat on the editorial board of another antibiotics-related publication, whose research articles had been cited in the ad created by William Douglas McAdams for the antibiotic Sigmamycin—the same ad that featured the business cards for doctors who didn't exist. Welch had cited Sigmamycin when, as an FDA official, he heralded the dawn of a new era of increased antibiotics use.

The Sacklers never spoke to Lear, and he was unable to find the final link tying them to MD Publications. The thicket of corporate paperwork and tangled business dealings surrounding MD Publications was just too dense to penetrate. If Lear had proved his case, the carefully constructed world of Arthur Sackler might have tumbled down in 1962. As it was, Arthur and his brothers soon left John Lear behind.

By the 1970s, Purdue Frederick, though still small, was a very profitable business and had made Mortimer and Raymond Sackler extremely wealthy. Purdue hit a home run when in 1966 it acquired a line of antiseptic products sold under the brand name Betadine, one of which was the orange-colored disinfectant hospitals used to scrub down patients prior to surgery. For Purdue, it was an ideal product, with its low production costs and high profit margins. In 1969, Betadine even enjoyed a fleeting moment of fame when astronaut Neil Armstrong used the solution to decontaminate the Apollo landing module after his historic moonwalk.

The Sacklers' business operations had expanded overseas by the 1970s, and Mortimer and Raymond Sackler were living on different sides of the Atlantic. Raymond, who remained in Connecticut, became most closely associated with Purdue Frederick, the company's American arm. Mortimer was principally responsible for the family's European operations, including a British company called Napp Pharmaceuticals, essentially Purdue's English counterpart. Over time, the Sacklers would develop ties to pharmaceutical companies in Australia, Canada, Germany, and Japan. But it was Napp's acquisition of a Scottish drug producer, Bard Laboratories, that set the stage for the Sacklers' involvement in pain treatment.

Bard researchers had developed a sustained-release technology suitable for morphine. In 1980, Napp began to sell sustained-release morphine in England, under the brand name MST. Four years later, after more-rigorous testing required by the FDA, Purdue Frederick put the same drug on the market in the United States as MS Contin, the morphine-based predecessor to Oxy-Contin.

By that time, Mortimer and Raymond Sackler were sixty-eight and sixty-four years old, respectively. They would remain lifelong business partners, though by all accounts the two men had vastly different personalities and lifestyles. According to one mutual acquaintance, they sometimes clashed and during Purdue board meetings sat separated from each other by lawyers. Acquaintances frequently described Raymond as quiet and retiring. Mortimer was outgoing and loved the swirl of high society. He, like his older brother, Arthur, married three times, twice to far-younger women. Unlike Arthur, who was known even to his friends as a tightwad, Mortimer owned palatial homes in London, the English countryside, the French Riviera town of Cap d'Antibes, and an Austrian resort village in the Alps. During summer days on the Riviera, guests regularly arrived in the late afternoon to join Mortimer for backgammon on the villa's rear patio. A tennis coach was on staff to give lessons to the Sacklers and their guests. In winter the action moved to the Alps, where Mortimer hired skiing instructors. He lavished expensive gifts on his wives. In his second wife's vast collection of jewelry were two sets of Bulgari earrings valued at $480,000.

Mortimer's generosity extended beyond his wives and guests. Along with his brother Raymond he was a major donor to British art museums, including the British Museum, the Ashmolean Museum, the Serpentine Gallery, and other scientific and medical institutions. The Sackler brothers also gave large sums to various institutions in this country, including the Guggenheim Museum, the American Museum of Natural History, and the Smithsonian.

Mortimer Sackler might have had motives for residing in Europe beyond living the good life. During a bitter divorce battle, his second wife, Gertraud, or "Geri," as she was known, suggested in court papers that Mortimer's decision to leave the United States was driven by his decision to avoid paying taxes. Those papers stated:

> Mortimer D. Sackler, who was born in Brooklyn, New York, renounced his American citizenship in year 1974 and became a citizen of Austria and a resident of various countries in Europe. This was admittedly done by him to avoid paying United States taxes on his income in the United States as well as abroad.

Years later, Geri Sackler changed her story and said her former husband also felt a strong emotional tie to Austria because his parents had lived in Eastern Europe before immigrating to the United States. Whatever the reason, Arthur was apparently furious that his brother had given up U.S. citizenship. By the time OxyContin went to market in the mid-1990s, Mortimer had long been married to his third wife and spent most of the year living in London. He traveled to the United States only occasionally, to attend Purdue board meetings or art-world events.

• • •

ARTHUR SACKLER died in 1987. His memorial tribute was held at the Temple of Dendur at the Metropolitan Museum of Art. "He was a truly good person, a fine, splendid, noble human being with absolute integrity," his third wife, Gillian, said at the service. "He never had a small, devious, or petty thought."

During his later years, Sackler had sought to conquer the art world with the same determination that marked his business career. While making major donations to the Metropolitan Museum of Art, for instance, he used a museum storage room as a personal warehouse for his ever-growing collection of antiquities. Though he was a formidable collector, Arthur Sackler's quest for recognition as a cultural mandarin was never successful. One auction-house executive expressed his general opinion about Arthur by saying shortly after his death that "he had the charm of the dollar sign."

Arthur Sackler had spent his life keeping the family business dealings well hidden, and he expected, no doubt, that those secrets would follow him to the grave. But his death set off a brutal, nearly decade-long legal battle over his vast estate between Gillian, who was known as "Jill," and his four children. While his estate was valued in legal papers at $140 million, one of his former financial advisers estimated its worth at many times that amount. As Arthur's heirs fought over the spoils, some of the Sackler brothers' best-kept secrets, including their hidden business ventures, finally spilled out in court papers and into public view.

Arthur Sackler, for example, had long portrayed himself as a fierce competitor of Ludwig W. Frohlich, who ran the other dominant drug-advertising agency of the 1950s and 1960s. But court papers showed that the three Sackler brothers and Frohlich were collaborators and partners. In a memo Arthur Sackler wrote in 1973, he referred to "properties jointly built between myself, Mr. Frohlich and my brothers." Among those ventures was IMS Health, a prescription-tracking company that pharmaceutical companies use to learn about the drugs a doctor is prescribing, so that sales reps can tailor their pitches. Decades later, Purdue would use IMS data to identify doctors who were writing large volumes of OxyContin prescriptions or were likely to do so. As far as the public knew, Frohlich was the owner and head of IMS. But Arthur Sackler's children and lawyer claimed that the idea for IMS came from him, and that his brothers, Mortimer and Raymond, were also partners in the business.

At a meeting of the trustees of his estate, Arthur's lawyer and longtime confidant, Michael Sonnenreich, explained that "under the four-way agreement, [Arthur] gave away his rights to IMS. . . . But his understanding with Frohlich was that if he ever sold it, he was entitled to one-fourth." At the same trustees' meeting, Arthur's daughter Elizabeth railed at her uncles for cutting her father out of the money due him from IMS when the company went public. "Dad came up with the idea for IMS, and on a handshake with Bill Frohlich, Bill was given the go-ahead," she said, according to the minutes of that meeting. "I don't know a lot of the intermediary steps that happened, but I know that when Frohlich died, Raymond and Morty made out like bandits when the stock went public. As I understood it, Dad received nothing."

Jill Sackler also claimed that Raymond and Mortimer had helped themselves to profits from Purdue Frederick that should have gone to their older brother. "There was supposed to be a three-way agreement with Purdue Frederick, and they have taken gigantic sums out of that," she told Sonnenreich during another trustees' meeting. It fell to the lawyer to untangle a lifetime of business dealings between Arthur Sackler and his brothers. Long before the battle between Arthur's children and Jill Sackler was settled, a deal was struck under which Mortimer and Raymond agreed to pay the estate $22,353,750 for their brother's one-third stake in Purdue.

John Lear, the journalist who had tried to penetrate the Sacklers' empire, died in 1999, unaware that these court documents existed. Had Lear had the chance to sort through them, he would have discovered that much of what he had suspected about Arthur Sackler and his brothers was right. The documents in Arthur Sackler's estate indicated that the Sackler brothers owned MD Publications, the company that funneled some $260,000 in payments to Henry Welch, the disgraced FDA official, by disguising those funds as reprint royalty fees. The ownership of MD Publications had bounced around, but the documents indicated that Mortimer and Raymond Sackler—or entities controlled by them— were the two mysterious unidentified stockholders in the business. The final resting place for MD Publications within Arthur Sackler's estate spoke loudly. As the top executive at Sackler's advertising firm had put it, "To me, the whole thing was Arthur."

By that time, Mortimer and Raymond Sackler were preparing OxyContin for its launch. Forty years had passed since they had started their pharmaceutical careers peddling l-Glutavite, the "metabolic cerebral tonic." Adversaries like John Lear had long ago been vanquished. They had amassed enormous wealth and given much of it to museums and medical institutions. The Sackler name was now engraved on cultural and educational temples throughout the world.

Arthur Sackler had been an original and a visionary. But as reports of OxyContin abuse mounted, Mortimer and Raymond, now in their golden years, faced a threat to their reputations and legacy. It was a challenge that would have tested their brother's abilities.

FOUR

A Pot of Gold

IN AUGUST 2000, A LETTER LANDED ON ART VAN ZEE'S DESK. It was an invitation to an upcoming meeting of a group called the Appalachian Pain Foundation. Van Zee hadn't heard of the organization, but it was clear from the enclosed material that its mission was to advocate the aggressive use of opioids in patients with chronic pain.

In the cover letter, a physician named Susan Bertrand quoted a seventeenth-century English apothecary, Thomas Sydenham, who wrote: "Among the remedies which it has pleased Almighty God to give man to relieve his suffering, none is so universal or efficacious as opium." Bertrand described herself as the founder of the Appalachian Pain Foundation and said its mission was to spread new medical thinking about treating pain more aggressively, through a series of educational meetings for doctors. The talks' sponsor was Purdue Pharma, manufacturer of OxyContin.

By the time that letter arrived, Van Zee felt as though a lifetime of work trying to improve the health of people in Lee County was being swept away. There had always been a few patients abusing one pill or another. But now it was a rare day when he wasn't pulled aside by someone seeking help for a loved one whose desperate addiction to OxyContin had destroyed a family, financially or emotionally.

In Dryden, the tiny community where Van Zee lived, the son of one of his patients was shot dead, apparently while trying to steal OxyContin from a neighbor's house. In St. Charles, the town where he worked, escorts accompanied elderly women returning home from church to protect them from walking in on a burglar rifling through the medicine chest. Van Zee heard a parade of horror stories. Families saw their life's savings drained by a son or daughter's drug habit. Parents scoured pawnshops searching for family heirlooms hocked by an addicted child. The jail in Lee County swelled with young people arrested for drug-related crimes. Before long, the nephew of the local sheriff joined their ranks.

Van Zee would come home from work, eat a quick dinner, and then disappear downstairs into the basement. He and his son, Ben, once played a lot of Ping-Pong there. Now when his wife, Sue Ella Kobak, checked on her husband, she would find him sitting in his makeshift home office, scanning the Internet for news stories about OxyContin or swapping email messages with other doctors, addiction counselors, and newspaper reporters.

She began to worry. She knew her husband could withdraw into himself at times, even to the point of depression. Before their marriage, Van Zee had had a few long-term relationships with women, though none of them stuck. Then Sue Ella, a high-spirited and brassy woman, decided to make Art her cause. She was a child of Appalachia, who was born to activist parents and had followed in their footsteps. In the 1960s she had worked in the antipoverty program known as Volunteers in Service to America, or VISTA, where she also met her first husband, John Douglas Kobak. He had dropped out of Harvard University to come to Appalachia as a VISTA volunteer, but then he died suddenly in 1970 at the age of twenty-five, when Sue Ella was pregnant with their son, Zeke.

Sue Ella had long dreamed of becoming a lawyer—not just any type but one who would use the law to try to make Appalachia a little better. She entered law school at the University of Kentucky and, after graduation, went into practice as a community lawyer.

For a time, she and Art worked two sides of the same street. While he attended the sick, she took on coal companies and landfill operators on behalf of local community and environmental groups. She also worked as a public defender, representing those who couldn't afford a lawyer. She regularly bumped into Art and suggested he call her. He would quietly smile and say he might. He never did. A mutual friend suggested to both of them that they go out together. That didn't work either. Then one night in 1983, while at a restaurant with friends celebrating a courthouse victory, Sue Ella caught sight of Art as he walked in. She was tipsy from champagne. "Why haven't you called me yet?" she demanded. Three weeks later, he did. They married in 1986, had a son, Ben, and adopted a daughter, Sophie Mae.

Family life had mellowed Art Van Zee. Though he remained dedicated to the St. Charles clinic, he'd begun taking days off to spend time with his kids. But now he was spending long hours in his basement office, reading about OxyContin's abuse. From what he could tell, the painkiller seemed to be taking a haphazard, irrational journey. Suddenly, newspapers in one city or town would carry reports about overdoses and arrests. Then, while that fire was burning, papers in another town hundreds of miles away from the first would begin to publish stories about the drug. By mid-2000, Van Zee had learned that the painkiller's abuse was occurring not only in Virginia and Maine but also in Florida, Louisiana, Ohio, Pennsylvania, North Carolina, and even Alaska. A law-enforcement official in New Orleans told a newspaper there that OxyContin was being discovered by people who had abused traditional painkillers such as Vicodin as well as by heroin addicts. "This probably will be your new Vicodin," that drug agent was quoted as saying. "Many of our Vicodin abusers are just learning about it. Heroin addicts are starting to use it."

Van Zee belonged to a local group called the Lee Coalition for Health, which began meeting to try to figure out how to deal with the county's growing OxyContin crisis. Its other members included Vince Stravino, drug-abuse counselors such as Beth Davies, and law-enforcement officials, including the sheriff of Lee County, Gary Parsons.

Stravino was convinced that a public-health catastrophe was unfolding. He saw how the word about OxyContin's pure and powerful high was spreading through the grapevine from one satisfied user to another. It had happened that way with other prescription drugs that caught on with abusers. But with OxyContin, Stravino believed, the dangers were far greater. Oxy-Contin, because of its supercharged strength, was far less forgiving. As more people experimented with it, a lot of them wouldn't be able to walk away. Instead, they would get addicted, get hurt, or die.

Stravino wanted the Lee Coalition to apply pressure on the Food and Drug Administration to remove the painkiller from the market. The drug had already created more damage than some medications that the FDA had recalled in the past, he argued, and there were other painkillers that doctors could use that posed fewer risks.

At the time, Van Zee thought otherwise. The drug worked for some of his patients and he wasn't ready to call for its removal. Still, while doing his Internet research, he had found issues that deeply troubled him. Primary among them was the nature and scale of Purdue's marketing campaign. Company sales reps were handing out to doctors and nurses promotional gifts such as stuffed animals and beach hats emblazoned with OxyContin's logo, or a compact disc entitled *Swing Is Alive*, which featured songs such as the Andrews Sisters singing "Boogie Woogie Bugle Boy." The photograph on the recording's cover showed an older couple dancing, apparently free of arthritic pain thanks to Oxy-Contin.

Van Zee knew that drug companies routinely gave out such gifts when promoting a new product. But he was disturbed that Purdue was employing the same strategies used to promote a blood-pressure or cholesterol treatment to sell an extremely powerful narcotic. It seemed particularly ill-advised given the painkiller's widening abuse.

Van Zee's style wasn't to point fingers. He assumed that the doctors and scientists working at Purdue were well intentioned and that their aim was to help people, not hurt them. If anything, he thought, company officials were probably unaware of the problems that OxyContin was causing in places like Lee County, and he figured that if he could connect with someone at the company, a fellow doctor perhaps, they could work together to get the crisis resolved.

Van Zee didn't know anybody at Purdue. But a Purdue physician, J. David Haddox, had appeared frequently in newspaper articles about OxyContin's abuse, defending the drug and Purdue's practices. Van Zee sent him a letter to request a collaboration:

> The extent and prevalence of the problem is hard to
> over-emphasize. . . . These problems are enormous ones
> for a poor rural area such as ours with minimal re-

sources for dealing with treatment and recovery of hard core narcotic addiction. This also presents an enormous challenge to all in the pain management community, as well as to the Purdue Frederick Company. I would look forward to having a dialogue with you further about this.

David Haddox, tall and fit, with a beard and a downturned mouth, held an impressive array of medical and professional credentials. He first went to dental school but, upon completing that degree, he decided to become a doctor. He went to medical school and received training in pain management, addiction medicine, and psychiatry.

During the early 1990s, he headed the pain-management department at Emory University School of Medicine and also served as the head of the American Academy of Pain Medicine. Unlike Russell Portenoy, Haddox was not a trained researcher, but he became one of the pain-management movement's most vocal advocates. He coined a catchphrase, "pseudoaddiction," which opioid advocates embraced. Haddox and a coauthor first used the term in a 1989 paper to describe a situation in which a doctor might mistakenly identify a patient exhibiting the signs of compulsive drug-seeking behavior—going to multiple doctors for prescriptions, for instance—as a drug addict. But Haddox argued that such behavior might be a "pseudoaddiction" and actually reflect the plight of a patient who was receiving inadequate medication to treat their pain. The solution, Haddox and his coauthor wrote, was to treat such patients with more opioids.

Haddox's argument wasn't based on a study involving hundreds of patients or even a dozen of them. Instead, it was a theory that Haddox based on his analysis of a single patient's behavior. But opioid advocates and drugmakers such as Purdue Pharma embraced "pseudoaddiction" as a legitimate concept, because it fit neatly into their view that unwarranted fears about narcotics were causing pain patients to suffer.

It also apparently helped land Haddox a job with Purdue. He had tried unsuccessfully to find a position in the pharmaceutical industry, until a Purdue executive approached Haddox after he gave a talk in 1999. He was soon the company's public point man on the issue of OxyContin abuse, a position that gave him a high-profile platform not only to air his strong views about pain care but also to exercise his often-combative personality.

In early 2000, soon after the U.S. Attorney in Maine, Jay McCloskey, alerted physicians about the growing problems with addiction to OxyContin, a reporter at a small newspaper in southwestern Virginia received a call from Haddox. The newspaper, the *Richlands News Press*, had started running articles about an explosion of OxyContin abuse in Tazewell County, Virginia, which is near the West Virginia border about a hundred miles northeast of Pennington Gap. Haddox called the reporter who wrote these articles, Theresa M. Clemons, and told her he wanted to help her put issues about OxyContin into perspective.

In a subsequent article, Clemons quoted Haddox as saying that while misuse or abuse of drugs like OxyContin did occur, such problems were minor compared with the lack of proper pain treatment. He also emphasized that powerful painkillers like OxyContin posed little addiction threat to patients. "If you take the medicine like it is prescribed," he said, "the risk of addiction when taking an opioid is one half of one percent."

For Purdue, publicity about OxyContin's abuse came at an awkward time. By 2000, the drug was a blockbuster, with annual sales of $1 billion and seemingly unlimited prospects for future growth. The painkiller was transforming once-sleepy Purdue into an emerging giant, and OxyContin sales now accounted for 80 percent of the company's soaring revenue. But by 2000, Purdue also knew that federal drug agents were investigating several doctors in Virginia and elsewhere for illegally prescribing OxyContin and other narcotics. Other physicians had pulled back from prescribing it in response to a growing stream of newspaper articles covering abuse of the drug. OxyContin also had a new nickname. It was called "hillbilly heroin."

In response to the bad press, Purdue executives, working with Susan Bertrand, launched the Appalachian Pain Foundation. Even before the organization was formed, Bertrand was being paid by Purdue to give speeches to doctors and druggists about pain management, including one she gave in early 2000 at a pharmacy school. Several Purdue sales representatives were present and Bertrand met with them after it. She described her concerns about the growing abuse of OxyContin and how it might negatively affect the ability of patients to get the drug. She offered to set up a group that would advocate for the use of Oxy-Contin and other strong narcotics and help doctors better understand how to use them. The Purdue representatives welcomed the plan and said the company would pay for all the organization's costs, such as renting meeting halls.

In September 2000, several Purdue executives, including David Haddox, arrived in Charleston, West Virginia, for the Appalachian Pain Foundation's kickoff meeting, which was billed as a pain-treatment seminar for local doctors. Before it started, Haddox and others met briefly with a contingent of officials from Tazewell County, the area featured in the *Richlands News Press* articles. A local prosecutor, Dennis Lee, painted a vivid picture of the devastating toll that OxyContin misuse was taking in terms of addiction and crime. Haddox and his colleagues appeared sympathetic but told Lee that the problems in places like

Tazewell County were isolated incidents and reflected the depressed economies in those areas and a long history there of using narcotic painkillers to treat injuries caused by occupations like farming, mining, and logging. Lee walked away from the discussion feeling that Haddox and his Purdue colleagues had failed to grasp the severity of the crisis that was unfolding.

About a month later, the Appalachian Pain Foundation held a meeting in Richlands, Virginia, a town two hours from Pennington Gap. Haddox was again the event's main speaker and Art Van Zee saw the meeting as an opportunity to meet him, so he, Beth Davies, and Elizabeth Vines piled into Van Zee's car and drove there. During his talk, Haddox emphasized that doctors needed to take precautions when prescribing drugs like OxyContin, including monitoring a patient's use of such pills and keeping accurate records. As Van Zee listened, he realized that the Purdue executive, despite his sensible warnings, had come to southwestern Virginia to promote the greater use of OxyContin at a time when its abuse was already out of control. Dennis Lee, the prosecutor, was also there, and he and Van Zee spoke during a panel discussion about the catastrophes affecting their communities.

"We have never seen anything like this before," Lee said. "There is just no comparison."

Van Zee approached Haddox and introduced himself as the doctor who had written to him. He commended Purdue for wanting to reduce the misuse of its drug, but he told Haddox he was concerned that the company was still sending out promotional gimmicks like the Swing Era music CD.

"How is that any different from what every other drug company does?" Haddox asked him.

"People aren't stealing from their families or breaking into their neighbors' homes over blood-pressure pills," Van Zee replied.

Haddox excused himself, saying he had a long drive ahead. He was scheduled to give a talk the following morning at a meeting of the Appalachian Pain Foundation in eastern Kentucky, another area rife with OxyContin abuse. He suggested that Van Zee direct his complaints elsewhere.

"I don't have anything to do with that," Haddox told him. "This is a marketing-department issue."

The marketing genius of the Sackler family, Arthur Sackler, was long dead when OxyContin appeared. But the strategies that Purdue used to position and promote the drug were as ambitious as any he might have devised. From the beginning, company executives planned to turn OxyContin into the first powerful narcotic ever mass-marketed for common conditions such as lower-back pain, arthritis, surgical pain, fibromyalgia, dental pain, and pain resulting from broken bones, sports injuries, and trauma. Simply put, the company's plan was to expand the use of long-lasting opioids from cancer wards into the mainstream of medicine by convincing thousands of family doctors, general practitioners, dentists, and anyone else who held a prescribing pen that OxyContin was safe and wouldn't lead to abuse and addiction by patients.

In 1995, a market research company hired by Purdue to interview doctors reported back that physicians were in "universal agreement" about wanting an opioid they could prescribe "without the concern regarding side effects or addiction." They also responded favorably when told that a new long-acting narcotic produced fewer "peaks and valleys" than a traditional painkiller in a patient's blood. The marketing firm, Groups Plus, noted some physicians worried that a pure, long-acting narcotic might be "more susceptible to abuse." But Purdue knew that for Oxy-Contin to succeed it had to give doctors what they wanted, not what they feared, even if that meant creating illusions or having to lie.

Its unwitting accomplice in that campaign was the FDA. When the FDA approved OxyContin for sale in late 1995, regulators let the company make a claim for the drug that agency officials have never allowed for any other drug before or since. The FDA permitted Purdue to imply that OxyContin might pose a lower risk of abuse than traditional painkillers because it was a time-release narcotic. In the hands of Purdue, that hedged statement became a marketer's dream and a claim for OxyContin's safety.

The FDA reviews data about the safety and effectiveness of a drug for years prior to approving it for sale, and Purdue had pushed regulators during that process to authorize the company to make a variety of claims for OxyContin. In one 1993 submission, for instance, it laid out its argument about why it believed that a time-release drug would be less prone to abuse than standard painkillers. The company stated:

> A controlled-release formulation of oxycodone may have less abuse potential than drugs such as Percodan for several reasons. First, most illicit drug abusers prefer a drug that is rapidly acting. The controlled-release formulation will have a longer acting effect without producing an immediate euphoria. In addition, the tablet formulation of the controlled-release oxycodone will be more difficult to dissolve in a solution, hence not desired by the "street" addict, who prefers an injectable solution. Second, the controlled-release formulation of oxycodone will not be targeted for patients who might

otherwise be treated with codeine [a painkiller with less abuse potential than oxycodone] as has been the case [by some makers of oxycodone-containing drugs like Percodan] in the past. As previously stated, this controlled-release formulation of oxycodone will be useful in the treatment of patients with acute or chronic moderate to moderately-severe pain.

This all made sense on paper, but Purdue never put any of it to the test by running studies to determine, for example, whether drug abusers might actually prefer OxyContin to traditional narcotics. The FDA accepted it, nonetheless, relying on studies that proved meaningless when OxyContin hit the streets.

One of those reports was published in 1993 in the respected *Journal of General Internal Medicine*. It was conducted by a researcher, Dr. Daniel Brookoff, who interviewed 130 hospital patients with a history of abusing prescription narcotics. About 85 percent of those patients told Brookoff they had tried to abuse time-release painkillers and, of that group, the majority said they had found that time-release narcotics such as MS Contin were of "little or no use" from an abuser's perspective. They also speculated that such painkillers would have little value on the street, Brookoff reported. "These results suggest that controlled-release narcotic formulations may have a lower potential for abuse than do other narcotic medications," Brookoff wrote in the study's conclusion. "In situations where there is concern about potential abuse or diversion of prescribed narcotics, controlled-release preparations may be an appropriate alternative to high-peaking, rapid-onset opioid formulations."

The FDA required Purdue to provide warnings on information about OxyContin for doctors and patients, similar to those used for MS Contin. Among other things, that language warned

that breaking, chewing, or crushing a tablet could release a "potentially toxic" dose of narcotic and that the risk of overdose
from the drug was particularly acute for so-called "opioid naïve"
patients, or those who had not taken narcotics before. The drug's
label also noted that oxycodone-containing painkillers were
"common targets for both drug abusers and drug addicts."

But the claim that the FDA allowed Purdue to make for Oxy-
Contin trumped all those warnings and soon became the linch-
pin of the company's massive marketing campaign. It read:
"Delayed absorption, as provided by OxyContin tablets, is believed to reduce the abuse liability of a drug." Prior to OxyContin's approval, regulators had debated whether to allow Purdue
to make the claim. The FDA examiner who managed the drug's
review, Curtis Wright IV, supported it, arguing that if one was
concerned about a narcotic producing a sense of euphoria in a
patient, it was right to use a medication that built up in the
bloodstream "more slowly . . . and is not given very frequently."

But in November 1995, a month before OxyContin's approval,
another FDA official, Diane Shnitzler, challenged the notion of
including the language in the drug's label. "Sounds like B.S. to
me," she wrote Wright. "Any truth to this statement or legit reason to be in label?"

"Actually, Diane, this is literally true," he responded. "One important factor in abuse liability determination is how fast the
'hit' is from a drug, as this has marked effect on 'high' . . . Oxy-
Contin cooked up and injected no, oral tablets taken by mouth
are probably less desirable than percodan."

A month later, when OxyContin was approved with a label
containing a claim suggesting lower abuse, there was celebra-
tion inside Purdue. In an internal report, Purdue executives
touted the FDA-approved language as "so valuable and promotional that it could have easily served as [OxyContin's] principal

selling tool." In 1998, Curtis Wright joined Purdue as an executive medical director with a first-year compensation package worth $379,000 in salary, bonuses, and other benefits.

As sales of OxyContin began, Purdue's marketing department devised strategies to reinforce the message sounded by opioid advocates: that millions of Americans were suffering needlessly from pain because of outdated stigmas about narcotics and their safety. In one marketing document, a Purdue executive proposed conducting a survey about untreated pain, which could be distributed to the news organizations. He wrote:

> In an effort to create a "media hook" that would coincide with the launch of OxyContin, a consumer survey conducted by a company such as The Gallop Poll is being proposed. This survey would focus on the prevalence and problems of chronic pain, both malignant and non-malignant. The release of the results of such a survey would be publicized along with the recent FDA approval of a new controlled-release Oxycodone preparation: OxyContin. This is a classic problem/solution strategy to create a need for the launch of a product such as OxyContin.

It's not clear whether that survey was conducted, but a later one underwritten by Purdue found the problem of chronic pain to be one of staggering scope. Its key "finding": that at least one family member in 44,000,000 households nationwide—or nearly one-half of the homes in the United States—suffered from chronic pain.

"Why does this suffering continue?" a publicity release asked. "Underuse of opioids (narcotics), such as morphine and codeine, is one reason."

Sales of OxyContin during its first two years on the market were relatively low-key. During those years, Purdue began to build its own large network of sales reps to market the drug to doctors and hospitals, and initially it forged a deal in 1996 with Abbott Laboratories, a much bigger pharmaceutical company, to help promote the drug.

Purdue intended to completely transform how doctors treated the pain of common problems such as back pain, arthritis, and injuries by convincing them to switch to OxyContin from other narcotic painkillers and even from pain drugs that did not contain narcotics. But first the company needed to convince physicians that they were not adequately treating pain and that OxyContin was the answer to that problem because it was more convenient, safer, and less likely to addict their patients than traditional painkillers.

To launch its campaign, Purdue sent invitations to doctors, urging them to attend all-expenses-paid meetings at resort locations in Arizona, California, and Florida. The theme of those gatherings was the "undertreatment" of pain in the United States and its solution: more-aggressive prescribing of long-acting narcotics such as OxyContin. Over time, between two and three thousand doctors would attend those junkets. Purdue also used these events to recruit hundreds of doctors for its "speakers bureau," a term for the roster of physicians paid by pharmaceutical companies to give talks to medical professionals. Purdue was not the only company that sponsored "educational" junkets for doctors or paid physicians to pitch products to their colleagues. Every drug manufacturer was doing so. The practices were testimony to both Arthur Sackler's work to unify the financial interests of drugmakers and doctors and a delusion among physicians that industry payments to them were not a form of influence-peddling.

Some of Purdue's speakers, like Dr. Susan Bertrand of the Appalachian Pain Foundation, got $500 per talk. Better-known pain experts earned upward of $3,000. Purdue's speakers appeared at a variety of venues, including staff meetings at hospitals, events at local medical societies, and continuing-education programs for nurses, pharmacists, and others. By Purdue's own estimate, it sponsored thousands of these talks in the years following the launch of OxyContin. The company had sponsored similar events when it first sold MS Contin, which were attended by cancer specialists and pain experts. But the audiences for talks that introduced OxyContin were different. They were comprised of physicians who lacked training in both managing pain and recognizing patients prone to drug abuse.

Purdue insisted that these presentations were intended only to raise medical awareness about the inadequacy of pain treatment rather than to market OxyContin. But the number of competing pain-relieving drugs could be counted on a few fingers, and company officials were well aware that their presentations invariably promoted OxyContin. Purdue's 1998 budget included a push "to convince health care professionals (physicians, nurses, pharmacists, and managed care professionals) to aggressively treat both non-cancer pain and cancer pain. The positive use of opioids, and OxyContin tablets in particular, will be emphasized."

Traditionally, doctors prescribed long-acting painkillers such as OxyContin only after milder ones had failed. But Purdue wanted to convince doctors to use OxyContin before trying weaker medications such as "combination" drugs—those like Percocet and Tylox, which mixed a narcotic with an over-the-counter pain reliever—or a non-narcotic painkiller called Ultram. Also in the budget for 1998 was a directive "to convince MDs to prescribe, as well as RNs and appropriate pharmacists to recommend, OxyContin Tablets for both opioid-naïve or opioid-exposed patients with moderate-to-severe pain lasting more than a few days instead of combination opioids and Ultram and, through proper dosing and [dosage adjustment], eliminate or delay the need for other long-acting opioids."

The marketing of OxyContin was the most ambitious undertaking in Purdue's history. By 1998, the company's sales force stood at about 625 people, about twice the level prior to the drug's introduction, and about 70 percent of those sales reps were assigned to sell OxyContin. Each new salesperson hired received three weeks of company training, with four days specifically devoted to MS Contin and OxyContin. The programs, conducted at Purdue headquarters, included presentations on the history of pain care, its science, and the company's mission to better it. Sales reps were also schooled in the basics of pain medicine from the perspective of opioid advocates. During training, they were quizzed on lessons learned, including one question concerning the risk of addiction posed when a doctor prescribes a narcotic to a patient, or so-called iatrogenic addiction. The required answer was always the same: "less than one percent."

After training, each sales rep went out into the field to work a specific geographic territory, under the supervision of a district area manager. Purdue equipped its reps with the most modern pharmaceutical marketing tools available. Like other drugmakers, the company worked with IMS Health, the prescription-data-collection company—in which the Sackler family once held a hidden interest. IMS data told Purdue reps not only how much OxyContin a particular doctor was prescribing but also how many prescriptions were written for competing painkillers. An internal company site updated IMS data as soon as new statistics were available. Purdue marketing officials massaged this data into reports and placed them on the same site, under names such as Outlet Zip Report, Core Coverage Report, and Combo Opportunity Report. The "opportunity" in the Combo Opportunity Report was a reference to doctors who were good sales targets because they were already prescribing high volumes of combination drugs like the painkillers Percocet and Vicodin. In Purdue's marketing lingo, doctors were ranked, according to their prescribing volume, as "decibels," with a decibel 10 indicating the highest volume. Doctors classified at between 8 and 10 were considered prime opportunities.

In making their pitches, Purdue reps pointed to OxyContin's longer-lasting action and purity as advantages over traditional painkillers. But company reps continued to face a major hurdle—convincing doctors leery about narcotics that their patients wouldn't get addicted to OxyContin or abuse the drug. A survey of doctors prior to the drug's launch indicated that it might be doomed to be a niche product used only for patients in severe pain. But when the FDA allowed Purdue to claim that OxyContin might be less prone to abuse than traditional painkillers, it gave sales reps a powerful tool. One training memo about how to present OxyContin to doctors was entitled "If I Only Had a Brain . . ." It read:

> In The Wizard of Oz, Dorothy had a clear-cut objective. She knew exactly what she wanted—to get back home to Kansas. Who could help her? Only one person could give her what she wanted: The Wizard. According to the munchkins, the Right Approach (how to accomplish this task) was to take the Yellow Brick Road. The attention-grabber was Dorothy's painting-the-picture of her Auntie Em. Turns out that Dorothy knew that the guard also had an Auntie Em. That got them inside.

Toto eventually grabbed the Wizard's attention by pulling down his curtain. Then Dorothy knew she had to "ask" for his attention.

The memo went on:

Know your listener and his/her needs/wants: Gather facts about your customer prior to your call. Firing at a target in the dark is not very promising. As you prepare to fire your "message," you need to know where to aim and what you want to hit! "The physician wants pain relief for these patients without addicting them to an opioid."

Have a Well-formulated Approach: A single thought or sentence that will best lead you to your objective. "According to the FDA, stated in the OxyContin package insert, 'Drug addiction is characterized with the procurement, hoarding and abuse of drugs for non-medicinal purposes.' 'Delayed absorption, as provided by OxyContin tablets, is believed to reduce the abuse liability of a drug.'"

The memo closed: "A pot of gold awaits you 'Over the Rainbow'!"

Recruiting sales reps to sell OxyContin was never a problem for Purdue, because the company's bonus system was among the most lucrative in the pharmaceutical industry. Typically, the bonus paid to a sales rep is based on the increase in the number of prescriptions the doctors in a rep's territory write for a company's products from one year to another. Purdue's system was based instead on an increase in the dollar value of OxyContin prescribed. As a result, Purdue sales reps had a financial incentive to encourage doctors to prescribe higher dosages of Oxy-Contin: The higher the dose per pill, the more it cost.

This system had another predictable result. Some of Purdue's highest-paid sales reps worked areas where doctors operated illegal pill mills and OxyContin abuse was rampant. One of these "hot spots," as Purdue called them internally, was the resort town of Myrtle Beach, South Carolina. Local drugstore owners told Purdue sales reps there that suspicious "patients" were traveling to an area pain clinic to get OxyContin. From morning to night, dozens of cars—many of them with out-of-state license plates—jammed the parking lot of a strip mall where the clinic was located.

One Myrtle Beach druggist, Ron Mason, said he confronted a local Purdue sales rep soon after his own pharmacy had been robbed for the second time. During the first holdup, which took place in 1999, a thief had entered the store, put a gun to the head of an employee, and demanded OxyContin by name. Mason believed the rep had to know what was going on at the local pain clinic but was silent because he was getting his commission on sales.

Even as DEA agents began to investigate the Myrtle Beach clinic, the value of OxyContin prescriptions written in the area boomed. In the first three months of 2001, sales grew by $1 million, which was $300,000 higher than the growth during that period for any other sales territory in the United States. When asked by a reporter about the huge increase, a Purdue spokesman attributed the boom to the large number of senior citizens living in Myrtle Beach who had conditions like arthritis that required pain medication.

Traditionally, makers of narcotics have not promoted their drugs directly to patients through consumer advertisements. But Purdue used other means to get the message about OxyContin out to patients. One way was through an existing public-relations program called Partners Against Pain; its website provided patients with referrals to pain specialists in their area. Purdue placed pamphlets and videotapes in doctors' waiting rooms, encouraging patients to talk with physicians about pain.

Some companies would have embraced the ability to legally claim that its drug might be less prone to abuse than those of competitors. But for Purdue, that wasn't enough. All over the country, the company's army of sales reps began promoting the drug to doctors, claiming either that it was less prone to abuse than traditional painkillers or that it couldn't be abused at all.

A sales rep in Indiana described OxyContin to a doctor as safer than traditional painkillers such as Percocet. A rep in South Carolina told a doctor that OxyContin was not addictive. And in Pennington Gap, a Purdue sales rep walked into a drugstore and assured a pharmacist named Greg Stewart that "drug abusers won't be interested in it."

FIVE

Senior Night

By the fall of 2000, Pennington Gap's tiny downtown strip was crowded with Oxy dealers. They stood on every corner, holding up either two fingers, indicating that 20-milligram Oxys were for sale, or four fingers, which signified that the 40-milligram versions were available. Lindsay Myers was a regular customer along with her new boyfriend, Ray, a local mechanic eight years older than she was.

Their Oxy habit was costing them about $300 a day, and Lindsay quickly emptied her bank account. But she found another source of cash, a fireproof safe in her parents' bedroom. Lindsay knew where the key was hidden, so while she was alone in the house, she took the key and opened the safe. Two cans that looked like shaving-cream containers sat on one shelf. She picked one up and unscrewed the false bottom. Fistfuls of crumpled hundred-dollar bills were stuffed inside. "Oh yeah, thank you, God," she thought, as she pulled out bills. Soon she was stealing money from the safe on a regular basis. Then one day when she went to get the key, she discovered someone had moved it.

The cutoff of Lindsay's cash supply coincided with the Senior

Night football game at Lee High, a tradition that took place during the Generals' last home game of the season. At halftime, the name of each player or cheerleader graduating that year was announced over a loudspeaker. Accompanied by proud parents, each senior would then walk across the 50-yard line, to the applause of friends and neighbors.

Senior Night was Lindsay's night to shine. She was the graduating captain of the cheerleading squad. But earlier that day, while the other cheerleaders stood onstage in the high school auditorium at a pregame pep rally, stomping, dancing, and screaming at the top of their lungs, Lindsay felt like she had the flu. She hadn't had an Oxy for twenty-four hours and she had been running back and forth to the bathroom all day. She knew she wasn't going to feel right until she got an Oxy.

After the pep rally, she met up with Ray. He was out of money but promised to call his brother and beg him to wire $100 right away. As soon as he got the money, he told Lindsay, he would buy two Oxy 40s and bring one to her.

At the game a few hours later, Lindsay tried to cheer on the Generals as she fought off her nausea. When the halftime whistle blew, she scanned the stadium, hoping for a glimpse of Ray, but saw her parents instead, standing by the sidelines. It was a big night for them, and they looked happy and relaxed as they chatted with the other parents.

Then it was time to begin the procession. Lindsay heard her name boom over the stadium's public-address system. "Lindsay Myers is a senior and is the captain of the girls' varsity cheerleading team," the announcer said. "She is the daughter of Jane and Johnny Myers. She is seventeen years old." Jane and Johnny escorted a miserable Lindsay across the field. When they reached the other sideline, Lindsay pretended to be happy as her parents kissed her and told her how proud they were. As soon as they walked away, she anxiously searched the stands for Ray. Finally she saw him working his way down the stadium steps toward the field. He didn't make eye contact with her but kept walking toward a tunnel that ran underneath the stadium. Lindsay waited a few minutes before slipping away from the other cheerleaders to follow him. Ray was waiting in the tunnel, already high. He handed her a small cellophane packet with an Oxy 40 inside. She went into a nearby bathroom, crushed the pill with a tube of ChapStick, snorted the powder, wiped her nose, and ran back out onto the field.

All over Lee County, the OxyContin crisis had gotten worse. The number of children who had to be placed in foster care because a drug-addicted parent was neglecting them had doubled. A local methadone clinic estimated prior to opening that it would daily treat about fifteen patients addicted to opioids during its first twelve months of operation. Six months after the clinic opened its doors, it was treating 250 people a day, the vast majority of them addicted to OxyContin.

Inside Purdue, the alert issued by the U.S. Attorney in Maine, Jay McCloskey, set off alarm bells. In a hastily scribbled note, the company's top public-relations strategist, Robin Hogen, told a senior marketing official that Purdue needed "a strategy to contain this!" At McCloskey's urging, the company agreed to end the weekend "educational" retreats it had been holding for doctors and also began to distribute prescription pads that couldn't be duplicated in copying machines or easily forged.

These steps seemed admirable but ineffectual to Art Van Zee. Purdue had set the OxyContin epidemic into motion, he believed, by radically expanding its market. If that was going to be undone, Van Zee believed, there would have to be dramatic changes in how Purdue marketed and sold the drug.

In November 2000, Van Zee reached out to David Haddox at

Purdue. A month had passed since their meeting in Richlands, and Haddox was planning another trip to the area. He agreed to meet Van Zee and a local drug-abuse counselor named Larry Lavender for dinner at a Holiday Inn near Pennington Gap.

OxyContin was by no means the first of its class to be abused. In fact, the history of narcotics had been a series of failed attempts to find a "magic bullet," a medication that would kill pain without becoming addictive. Morphine was initially considered less addictive than opium, and heroin was first marketed in 1898 as a less addictive substitute for morphine. Some physicians even championed heroin as a cure for morphine addiction, but its own allure quickly became evident, and heroin's manufacture was banned in 1924. A few years later, a new painkiller called Dilaudid, which contained a narcotic known as hydromorphone, was introduced. Hailed as a non-addicting substitute for morphine, Dilaudid was soon so widely abused it was nicknamed "drugstore heroin."

In the late 1960s, a pharmaceutical producer called Sterling Drugs announced that it had synthesized a drug called pentazocine, sold under the name Talwin, which had the painkilling properties of morphine but was non-addicting. These findings were based on a large test sample—thousands of people, including inmates at the federal prison facility in Lexington, Kentucky, tried the drug under supervision. And yet drug addicts soon discovered a way to get a heroin-like high from the medication. No one stood up to claim credit for the achievement, but cracking Talwin's defenses required ingenuity. By dissolving a tablet in water with a widely available antihistamine, you could create an injectable speedball that served as a heroin substitute known among addicts as "T's and Blues."

Within a few years, the abuse of Talwin had become so severe that Sterling decided to reformulate the drug by adding a compound called naloxone to it; the new drug was sold as Talwin NX. Like many narcotic painkillers, naloxone was also derived from the opium poppy, but it had an opposite effect to drugs such as heroin or oxycodone. Instead of stimulating "receptors," or neurotransmitters, in the brain and producing a high, naloxone blocked chemical transmissions at those sites, reversing the impact of a narcotic. Decades later, police officers would carry nasal sprays or hypodermic needles containing naloxone, also known as Narcan, in case they needed to revive someone who had overdosed. Adding naloxone to the Talwin didn't interfere with its painkilling properties, because when a pill was taken orally, as intended, the stomach neutralized the naloxone. But if an addict chose to shoot up Talwin NX, the naloxone blocked any high. Soon after Talwin NX appeared in the early 1980s, the drug's abuse dramatically declined.

Haddox was late, and when he finally arrived that evening at the Holiday Inn, he apologized and explained that he had just come from a community meeting in a North Carolina town dealing with OxyContin abuse. As the men dined, Haddox impressed Van Zee and Lavender with his knowledge of drug abuse and addiction. He responded sympathetically when Lavender told him a story about one of his patients, a thirteen-year-old girl, who was shooting up OxyContin intravenously. Over coffee, Van Zee raised his central concern that Purdue was making the drug too easy to get. Then he took out a sheet of paper from his jacket pocket, which contained a list of actions he wanted Purdue to take, and gave it to Haddox. It read:

1. Send a letter—red lettered—ALERT—to all physicians and mid-level practitioners calling attention to the fact that in some regions of the country there has been recognized large scale abuse of OxyContin

(used IV or snorted) leading to opioid dependence with the associated medical, personal, and social consequences usually seen with opioid addiction;

2. Send an even more extensive ALERT notice to all physicians practicing in pain management positions or specialties;

3. Stop marketing OxyContin for use in chronic non-malignant pain by stopping all advertisements that promote its use in this situation—i.e., chronic, non-malignant pain;

4. Revise Purdue Pharma's web site to reflect that there has been reported in some regions in the country extensive abuse of OxyContin, and give a detailed picture;

5. Stop sponsorship of pain management seminars around the country that promote heavily the use of opioids for chronic non-malignant pain;

6. Examine carefully the data that Purdue has concerning its sales of OxyContin in those regions of the country that we know have extensive abuse—specifically southwest Virginia; the Cincinnati, Ohio, area; the Altoona, Pennsylvania, area; and Maine.

Do these particular areas have a significantly higher prescribing pattern for physicians for OxyContin—i.e., in grams per 100,000 population area—are these areas where abuse is heavily seen, areas where there has also been much more frequent prescribing? etc.

Are these areas Purdue Pharma has chosen to market more heavily to physicians, etc. the use of OxyContin?

What other factors can we identify that would explain this kind of regional diversity in the abuse of the drug?

8. Replace OxyContin with Oxy/Nx—oxycodone/naloxone, which would presumably cut down substantially on the amount of abuse of the drug.

Art Van Zee, M.D.

After glancing at the document, Haddox assured Van Zee and Lavender that he would deliver the recommendations, and the three men wished each other good night. Heartened by Haddox's attention to the problem, Van Zee sent him a follow-up letter, thanking him for his time and again suggesting that Purdue consider funding educational programs about drug abuse in southwestern Virginia schools. Then he wrote a note to Dr. Daniel Spyker, another Purdue executive with whom he had been corresponding:

Larry and I appreciated meeting with David Haddox the other night. I appreciate very much David's time and interest in these issues of mutual concern. David had asked for some of my practical suggestions and I did give him a list written out on 11/20/00. Some of these may seem harsh and unrealistic. However, I don't think anyone ever would have imagined the scope and magnitude of abuse of OxyContin that is appearing in regions around the country. My fear is that these are sentinel areas, just as San Francisco and New York were in the early years of HIV [the virus that causes AIDS]. I don't think any of us understand all the reasons why this is occurring. Therefore, until this is better understood and

come to terms with, I do suggest these measures to stop
promoting OxyContin for use in chronic non-malignant
pain. I would think, until things are better understood
as to what is going on, that this would be in the best
interest of public health and Purdue.

Purdue had no interest in Van Zee's recommendations. But
not long after he gave them to Haddox, two drug-abuse experts
from Yale University, Dr. David Fiellin and Dr. Richard Schottenfeld, arrived at a community center in the tiny town of St.
Paul, Virginia, about fifty miles east of Pennington Gap. Nearly
150 people soon made their way into the hall, where a buffet-
style dinner—platters of chicken and biscuits and salad—was
laid out on tables. Many of those attending were doctors who,
like Vince Stravino, had come to work in Appalachia as physicians for the federal Public Health Service as a way of paying
back government loans for medical school.

Art Van Zee had arranged the meeting, for two reasons. He
hoped to educate physicians in and around Lee County who had
had little experience with opiate addiction. Heroin had never
been a substantial part of the drug scene in Appalachia. Places
like Pennington Gap were too far away from the big cities and
interstate highways that served as the hubs and trafficking routes
of the heroin trade. Now every doctor in the region was dealing
with people hooked on a legal drug, OxyContin, which was as
addictive as heroin. This medical community was particularly
vulnerable to the misinformation he believed was spread by
groups like the Appalachian Pain Foundation, and he hoped
good information would be an antidote.

Fiellin and Schottenfeld described for the crowd the process
of addiction and the different ways to treat it. Experts, they said,
don't know precisely why some people get addicted to a drug

and others don't and suspect that genetic, neurobiological, and social factors all play a role. There was a distinction, they pointed out, between addiction and drug dependency, the natural process in which a person taking an opioid under a doctor's supervision becomes physically, rather than psychologically, dependent on the drug. Opioid advocates had long argued that patients were being mischaracterized as addicts because they experienced withdrawal symptoms when the opioids they were taking were reduced or cut off. But some drug-abuse specialists believed that the lines between those two conditions were not so clear. The intense physical reaction and psychological stress caused by the withdrawal of a narcotic from a patient could play a role in the addiction. Put another way, if patients feared going through withdrawal, they would do what they could to stay on painkillers. Fiellin added that while he considered OxyContin an extremely useful medication, places like Lee County were not the best settings for prescribing it, because resources weren't available to deal with the calamities resulting from its misuse. Toward the meeting's end, one man in the audience confronted Van Zee and the Yale experts. He asked them if they thought the problem of opioid abuse would disappear if OxyContin was no longer prescribed. Later, someone told Van Zee that the man was a sales rep for Purdue.

In early December 2000, about a week after the meeting in St. Paul, Van Zee sat in his basement office, writing another letter, this time to the FDA. Initially he had felt upbeat after his meeting with David Haddox. But he had come to realize that whatever Haddox or any other Purdue official said, the company's actions—or rather its lack of action—spoke far more loudly about its intentions. A few days earlier, he had called the FDA headquarters in Rockville, Maryland, and told an official on the agency's controlled-substances staff about the scope of the OxyContin problem in southwestern Virginia. His letter, a follow-up to that conversation, described the outbreaks of Oxy-Contin abuse in Lee County and urged federal officials to take action. He also sent a copy to an official at another federal agency, the National Institute on Drug Abuse:

> This is a problem that is not being written about in the medical literature. The experts in the pain management community promote the use of opioids for chronic non-malignant pain and Purdue Pharma has marketed aggressively for the use of opioids in chronic non-malignant pain. The real life experience for the liberal use of opioids has proven to be a medical and social disaster for our region, and as I fear, may be a glimpse of what will happen nationally over the next few years.
>
> I would request that your office look into this further if at all possible. I could not over-state the major consequences this problem has had for our area.
>
> I have talked with Dr. Dan Spyker, senior medical director at Purdue Pharma. They are well aware of this problem. Among other things, I had suggested that a WARNING or URGENT NOTICE type of letter be sent to all physicians in the U.S. explaining that—at least in certain regions of the country—the OxyContin has been abused—snorted and injected—so as to lead to opioid dependence—and that all prescribing physicians need to be aware of this potential.

Soon afterward, Art Van Zee was making his rounds at Lee County Hospital when he ran into Vince Stravino. He told Stravino that he had been right. There was only one way to solve the OxyContin crisis and that was for the government to recall the drug. He hadn't come to that decision lightly. Purdue had forced his hand. The company had shown no interest in either taking steps he believed were critical in limiting the drug's availability or sending out an alert to doctors nationwide about the painkiller's increasing abuse. Van Zee had concluded that the company would never take responsibility for the troubles its painkiller was causing and would continue to market it as widely as possible.

He didn't want to start a battle with Purdue. But now he had no other choice. He and the people of Lee County would have to take a stand and convince the FDA it needed to act.

SIX

Hot Spots

IN MARCH 2001, A GROUP OF PURDUE EXECUTIVES ARRIVED in Richmond, Virginia, at the firm request of the state's attorney general, Mark Earley. Earley had written to Richard Sackler, Purdue's president—and Raymond Sackler's son—to say that he had "grave" concerns that the "widespread illegal sale of Oxy-Contin has created an epidemic of addiction and a surge in criminal behavior in Southwest Virginia."

The group of executives was led not by Richard Sackler but by the company's top lawyer, Howard Udell, who presented Earley with a plan similar to one the company had recently announced in Maine. It added provisions including a program to alert teenagers to the dangers of prescription drugs and a $100,000 grant to study the development of a prescription-monitoring system in Virginia.

Not long before, Van Zee had publicly announced a plan to hold a rally at Lee High to launch a citizens' petition asking the FDA to recall OxyContin. Purdue got wind of this plan and made it clear at the Richmond meeting that the company's offer to help financially support local drug-abuse-counseling programs had a string attached. The Lee County sheriff, Gary Parsons, who'd attended the meeting, relayed the news to Van Zee. Purdue didn't want Van Zee to have anything to do with those programs, Parsons told him, because the company was worried he would use its money to fuel his campaign against OxyContin. Van Zee didn't mind. "If it can help the county and I need to get left out, that's fine," he said.

A week later, at the Lee High auditorium, eight hundred distraught adults whose children, siblings, loved ones, or friends had been affected by OxyContin abuse filed in to hear Van Zee, and others, speak. Outside the school, a man clad in farmer overalls held up a hastily scrawled cardboard sign that read: TELL ON DRUG PUSHERS.

Jane Myers took a seat in the audience along with Lindsay and her boyfriend, Ray. It was Lindsay's first trip back to Lee High in two months. She and Ray were in rehab and, every day, they made a four-hour-long round trip between Pennington Gap and Knoxville, Tennessee, the site of the nearest methadone clinic. The facility was located in a rough part of Knoxville, and dealers stood on nearby street corners selling crack cocaine.

Lindsay was trying hard to stick with her methadone program. She couldn't attend classes at Lee High anymore, but her mother hired a teacher to tutor Lindsay at home every afternoon, so she would have a chance of graduating that spring with the rest of her class. Lindsay couldn't help feeling that in taking methadone she was trading one drug for another.

Van Zee and Beth Davies stood on the same stage Lindsay Myers had struggled across during the Senior Night pep rally. Sister Beth started the meeting, and several church leaders followed. Then Van Zee spoke. For a time, he said, he believed that OxyContin's benefits outweighed its risks. Now it was clear to him that its dangers were too great. "The pain and suffering brought to countless families and communities by the abuse of the drug surpass, by an extraordinary degree, its benefits," he said.

The *Powell Valley News*, a weekly published in Pennington Gap, gave most of the front page to its account of the meeting. The *News* also published Purdue's unequivocal response to the recall effort. In a letter to the editor, the drugmaker refused to recall OxyContin or place any limitations on its use. "Any effort to restrict access to OxyContin would be a disservice to the thousands of patients who rely on this medication to control their pain and regain function of their lives," the company said.

IT MIGHT seem odd that a billion-dollar drug company such as Purdue would bother responding to a small-town doctor like Art Van Zee. Officials such as David Haddox had spent 2000 traveling from one addiction-plagued community to another, insisting that the painkiller's abuse was limited to a number of "hot spots." And yet, by early 2001, company executives were beginning to see a powerful backlash against OxyContin. A massive drug raid in eastern Kentucky in February—dubbed OxyFest—in which more than two hundred people were arrested on charges of illegally possessing or selling OxyContin turned the drug's abuse from a local story into big news. Major media outlets seized on OxyContin as the tale of a "wonder" drug gone awry: a high-powered and reportedly abuse-resistant painkiller that had become a destructive street drug.

A few weeks after OxyFest, a lengthy front-page article in *The New York Times* raised questions about Purdue's safety claims for OxyContin and reported that some doctors and pharmacists believed the drugmaker had contributed to the problem by marketing it too aggressively. Coroners and other local authorities cited in the *Times* account estimated that OxyContin had been a factor in at least 120 drug-overdose deaths. One DEA official was quoted as saying that no other prescription drug introduced during the past two decades had been abused by so many so soon after going to market. Major articles about OxyContin abuse appeared in weekly newsmagazines including *Time*, *Newsweek*, and even *People*. A public-relations firm, FleishmanHillard, hired by Purdue to monitor news coverage of OxyContin reported that "OxyContin stories continue to permeate the media." Numerous examples were cited, including one 2001 report on the NBC television network that typified the tone of the media coverage. The public-relations firm wrote:

> On March 22, the NBC "Evening News" aired a segment focusing on the abuse of OxyContin among teenagers and young adults. While NBC's report provided fairly balanced coverage, it was led by a teaser on a number of local NBC affiliates, in some of the nation's biggest media markets, incorporating the story of a woman whose OxyContin-addicted husband tried to burn their house down. In her own words, "[T]hem things should be taken off the market. They are killing people." In the NBC "Evening News" national report, a physician said he won't prescribe OxyContin to his patients and suggests that the drug should be reformulated to make it less addictive. These statements . . . provide fire for legislators looking to regulate the prescribing patterns of physicians and, as a result of NBC's coverage, people all over the country heard them.

Before OxyContin, most journalists had never heard of Purdue Pharma. Nor was much known about the Sacklers. Even those who recognized the Sackler name were less likely to connect it with the pharmaceutical industry than with the art muse-ums, galleries, and medical schools underwritten by the family. Photographs of Sackler family members appeared occasionally in the society pages, but the family generally avoided any scru-tiny. Unlike most pharmaceutical companies in the United States, Purdue was privately owned by the Sacklers. Because its stock wasn't publicly traded, its financial records and business dealings were closed to outside inspection: Reporters didn't cover the company; drug-industry analysts didn't opine about its operations; and no outside directors, who serve on the boards of publicly traded companies, could influence it.

Even as the drugmaker faced an unprecedented crisis, the three members of the Sackler family most closely associated with Purdue—Mortimer, Raymond, and Raymond's son Richard—made no public comments about OxyContin's abuse. Instead, the Sacklers relied on Purdue executives such as David Haddox or the company's chief operating officer, Michael Friedman, and top lawyer, Howard Udell, to interact with government officials or the news media.

In early 2001, FDA officials, alarmed by published accounts of OxyContin abuse, contacted Purdue headquarters. According to one agency official, "It was made very clear to them that we were greatly concerned about what we were hearing and we wanted to know how we could work together and intercede before the problem got worse."

The fate of OxyContin and the fortunes of Purdue now hung in the balance. In 2000, Richard Sackler had told a gathering of sales reps that OxyContin's remarkable sales growth would continue to fuel the drugmaker for years to come. With the com-pany's reputation under attack and government regulators ques-tioning Purdue's response to the crisis, all of that was at risk.

Following the urging of Purdue executives such as Robin

Hogen, the company's chief public-relations officials developed several strategies to deflect criticism of its aggressive marketing of OxyContin and to avoid any restrictions on sales.

Purdue hired a small battalion of crisis-management experts and media consultants to supplement its small staff. One of them, the McGinn Group, had represented embattled breast-implant manufacturers and the lead-paint industry. Another firm, Nichols-Dezenhall, described itself as "the leader in crisis management and high-stakes communication." The two firms set out to calm the roiling waters surrounding OxyContin and to launch a counterattack against what Purdue officials felt were the media's unfair depictions of company practices. The counteroffensive that emerged was intended to reinforce the legitimate use of OxyContin, deflect the media's focus away from its abuse, and shift attention to the topic of prescription-drug abuse in general. As Purdue officials put it, OxyContin was simply the latest "drug du jour" in a long line of abused medications. To support their case, Purdue distributed pie charts intended to show that the number of overdose reports involving hydrocodone-containing painkillers like Vicodin was far higher than that involving oxycodone-containing drugs like OxyContin. These statistics, while not false, were misleading, because painkillers that contained hydrocodone were prescribed at three times the rate of those that contained oxycodone.

At the center of Purdue's defense was a sheaf of testimonies from satisfied pain patients. Company executives, after careful coaching by communications consultants, insisted publicly that it would be a tragedy if the behavior of drug addicts prevented legitimate patients from getting access to medication. In early 2001 a small Virginia public-relations firm, one of many local concerns hired by Purdue, described its mission as helping Purdue get "out the message that patients with pain are the 'silent victims' of all the press coverage of OxyContin abuse." Articles began to appear recycling a salvo from the early pain-management movement: that a new "war on drugs" threatened the well-being of pain patients. Some even argued that the news media's focus on OxyContin's dark side had exacerbated the abuse problem. One television critic, Tom Shales, suggested that the intense media coverage of OxyContin had inspired curious young people to experiment with the drug. News accounts, Shales wrote:

> tell you how to get high. Then the correspondents do follow-up reports expressing shock and dismay that the abuse is becoming more popular . . . Yeah, more kids are using the drug to get high because they heard about it and even saw how to use it on the evening news.

The growing coverage of OxyContin's abuse was having ripple effects, though they weren't what Purdue claimed. Some doctors reduced their prescriptions of OxyContin or stopped dispensing it altogether. And some patients asked doctors to take them off the painkiller even though they had been doing well on it.

David Haddox and other top executives at Purdue began meeting with newspaper editorial boards to present their case. Purdue, they said, had moved as quickly as possible to curtail OxyContin's abuse, launching an effort they described as without precedent in the pharmaceutical industry. The company had set what it described as a "new standard in corporate responsibility."

Purdue also launched a well-funded lobbying campaign aimed at convincing key members of Congress and officials of the Bush Administration that the company's "voluntary efforts to safeguard the use of OxyContin is the only effective means to proscribe it without interfering with the doctor-patient relationship," an internal Purdue report showed. One of the company's greatest fears was that the DEA would lower the limit on imports into the United States of thebaine, the opium-derived substance used to make OxyContin and other oxycodone-containing drugs.

"We were getting creamed; we were getting killed," Robin Hogen later told a gathering of corporate communications executives. "It was like being a prizefighter and you were getting punched in the stomach, and then in the cheek, and then in the stomach again, and you're sort of reeling. We were on the ropes with this kind of coverage on a product that creates about eighty percent of our revenue."

About a week after the rally at Lee High, Van Zee received a call from a Purdue staffer. She asked whether he would meet with a contingent of top company executives if they flew to Lee County to see him. Van Zee said he would be happy to do so. However, when he told Sue Ella about the phone call that evening, she expressed concern. Purdue hadn't told Art why they wanted to see him, and she worried that company officials planned to use the meeting to discuss the recall petition and maybe even threaten him with a lawsuit.

Years earlier, Sue Ella, while representing a local environmental group, had been sued for $10 million by a waste-disposal company that wanted to dump New York City garbage in Appalachia. The company's lawsuit, as well as its dumping plan, had failed. But she remembered how the company had used the lawsuit as a weapon to intimidate a much smaller opponent, and the lawyer in Sue Ella feared Purdue might try to use the same tactics against her husband. She told Art she didn't want him to go by himself to meet with the Purdue team, and when other members of the Lee Coalition for Health learned about the meeting, they agreed to go with him.

On a late March afternoon, three carloads of people left Pennington Gap and drove to a Ramada Inn in the nearby town of Duffield, Virginia. Along for the trip with Van Zee and Sue Ella were Beth Davies; Elizabeth Vines; Vince Stravino; Larry Lavender, the drug-abuse counselor; Greg Stewart, the pharmacist; and another man, who was a local bank official. When they entered the motel's lobby, a woman approached Beth Davies.

"Hello, Sister Davies," she said.

Davies didn't recognize the woman. "How do you know me?" she asked.

The woman explained that she worked for Purdue and had attended the Lee High meeting. She told the group that the company's corporate jet had been delayed taking off from Connecticut but that she expected her colleagues to land shortly.

They arrived an hour later. David Haddox shook hands with Van Zee and Lavender and then introduced his companions, including Purdue's chief operating officer, Michael Friedman, and its senior lawyer, Howard Udell. Udell was small and portly and, with a sagging double chin, looked older than his sixty years. He had spent much of his legal career working for the Sackler family, first through a New York City firm and later at Purdue itself. Udell could seem gracious and grandfatherly. But he was shrewd and aggressive, and he was playing a central role in trying to steer Purdue through the OxyContin crisis.

Friedman, tall with curly red hair and a mustache, had overall responsibility for Purdue's sales and marketing strategy. Before joining Purdue, he'd held top sales positions at an industrial-bolt manufacturer and a welding and metal-treatment business. According to a story that circulated around Purdue headquarters,

Friedman had found his way into the drug industry through a chance meeting with Richard Sackler on an airplane flight. Sackler was so impressed by his conversation with Friedman that he offered him a job. Initially, Friedman was responsible for seeking drug-licensing deals for Purdue, but he steadily worked his way up through the company. In the late 1990s, he became a top officer and announced at a company meeting that Purdue's growth would be so spectacular over the next decade that it would join the ranks of the ten largest drug companies in the United States.

As he shook hands with Van Zee and others at the Ramada, Friedman was conciliatory. "We understand you folks are having a horrible problem," he said. "We are here to see what we can do to help."

He began the meeting by describing the measures Purdue had already taken to cut down on OxyContin's misuse. Purdue had begun funding drug-counseling services in some areas and considered underwriting a similar program in Lee County. He took care to emphasize that Purdue would continue to offer such aid even if the Lee Coalition pursued its recall petition.

Friedman struck Van Zee and the others as courteous and concerned. But they were unmoved. If Purdue really wanted to help, they told him, the company should stop promoting Oxy-Contin for non-cancer pain until it was reformulated with naloxone. Purdue had recently announced that it was investigating ways to make the painkiller more resistant to abuse. But David Haddox responded that to simply withdraw it from the market without a replacement would harm patients who needed it.

The discussion went in circles until Stravino lost patience, telling the Purdue executives that neither he nor Van Zee had a stake in the OxyContin fight. Nobody in Lee County had anything to gain or lose from OxyContin either financially or professionally. They were only trying to stop a public-health calamity from spreading. Before long, Stravino warned, the poor, over-dosed sons and daughters of Appalachia turning up injured or dead in emergency rooms would be joined by kids from affluent suburban homes. Their parents wouldn't hesitate to sue Purdue, and the company would find itself embroiled in ugly, expensive litigation for years to come.

"The genie is out of the bottle," Stravino said. "This is only the beginning. This is going to follow you everywhere."

That was when Van Zee introduced the local bank official who had come with them to the meeting. He showed photographs of his family to the Purdue executives and talked proudly about his daughter, a successful teacher. Then he told Haddox, Udell, and Friedman a tale of the misery caused by OxyContin.

All the happiness had been squeezed out of his life, he said, after his youngest son became hooked on Oxys. It was a typical story. Things that could be easily sold, like tools and guns, began to disappear from the family's home. Then his son ran up huge credit-card bills. The boy denied he had a problem, even as he kept getting worse, until finally, when it seemed his life was in the balance, he agreed to seek help. Two years later, his son was barely hanging on. His OxyContin habit and ongoing treatment had already cost the family about $80,000, depleting the man's retirement savings. He told Friedman, Udell, and Haddox that he agreed with Van Zee. He thought Purdue should take the drug off the market until they could make it safer.

"We are an average American family," the man said. "Surely you have got enough patriotism to worry about this country?"

The Purdue group was silent. Finally, Friedman responded. "I'm sorry your family is having such a problem," he said.

Udell picked his briefcase off the floor and opened it. He removed several large pieces of paper and passed them around.

"I want to show you this because it's going to run in the local newspaper," he explained.

The pages were photocopies of a full-page newspaper advertisement. The ad's headline read: AN OPEN LETTER TO THE CITIZENS OF LEE COUNTY FROM PURDUE PHARMA. At its end, the "letter" bore David Haddox's name, as though it were a personal note from him. It read:

"I am a native of Appalachia and a physician who has spent much of my life studying and treating both pain and drug abuse. But today I am writing to you on behalf of Purdue Pharma L.P., the company that manufactures OxyContin Tablets." Haddox's letter went on to say that Purdue was greatly concerned about "the devastation that prescription drug abuse is having on Lee County" and was committed to addressing it. However, the company wanted to "clarify some information that was discussed at the recent meetings at Lee County High School so that we can work together from a platform of truth."

Some newspaper reports suggested that Purdue had placed a special emphasis on marketing OxyContin to doctors in poorer areas like Appalachia that relied on taxpayer-funded health-care programs like Medicaid. But the ad stated in boldface type that such claims were absolutely untrue. "It is equally false to say that Purdue knew about the abuse potential of OxyContin from the beginning and did nothing about it," stated the ad, which also disputed any suggestion that a reformulation of OxyContin would be quick or easy.

"We understand that Lee County residents are about to expend great effort and energy to promote a petition demanding the recall of OxyContin," the ad continued. "We are fortunate to live in a country where we can all express our views openly. However, we are concerned that the problem of abuse will not be solved by removal of a single drug, particularly one that millions of patients depend upon. . . . Instead of this futile petition drive, the energies of the people of Lee County could be spent on positive ways of dealing with the terrible problem of drug abuse and addiction." The ad suggested that this be accomplished through efforts including school education programs and prescription-monitoring plans.

To Stravino, Sue Ella, and Beth Davies, the purpose of the meeting was now clear. It was a setup orchestrated by Purdue to shove the ad down their throats. Furious, Sue Ella turned to Haddox.

"This is the most insulting thing that I have ever seen," she told him. "You have done more to hurt Appalachia than the coal industry has ever thought about doing."

Haddox sat bolt upright. "I resent that," he said.

"I don't give a damn if you do," she replied. "The truth will stand. I am not going to stay here."

She stormed out into the lobby. Greg Stewart, the pharmacist, soon joined her.

"I'm going to pay the bill," she told him.

"I've already paid it," he said.

"Did you pay for theirs too?" Sue Ella asked.

"Hell no," Stewart replied.

The following morning, the three Purdue executives met at a local café with Beth Davies and area officials, including Sheriff Parsons and Tammy McElyea, a county prosecutor. David Haddox still seemed to be sulking from the night before. Friedman and Udell listened as Sheriff Parsons and others described the way in which the area's law enforcement and drug-treatment programs had been overwhelmed by the abuse of OxyContin.

"Maybe we could help," Friedman offered.

"How much could you afford?" asked one official.

Friedman and Udell responded that the drugmaker would be

happy to contribute $100,000. Many at the table greeted the offer enthusiastically, but Sister Beth shot Udell a look.

The Purdue executives returned to Connecticut, where they apparently had second thoughts about the wisdom of the company's "open letter" to the people of Lee County, because it was never published. Meanwhile, the Lee Coalition for Health had to decide what to do about Purdue's offer. At a series of meetings, several members, including Sheriff Parsons and Greg Stewart, said they thought the group should accept the money. Stewart said that since Purdue had made a small fortune from the area's misery, it ought to give some of that fortune back to repair the damage. Van Zee was of a similar mind, and he drafted a letter from the coalition accepting Purdue's funds.

But Sister Beth told them it was blood money and that she would quit the coalition if they took it. She said she was sick of seeing corporate executives fly into Appalachia with their checkbooks as a way of buying peace. For years, companies from mining concerns to logging companies to garbage haulers and now a drug company had come to them with the same goal. Their executives all asked, "What can we do for you?" But what they really wanted was for their problems to go away.

This time, she insisted, they couldn't let that happen. Too many lives had already been destroyed. Yes, the money might do Lee County some good, but if they capitulated, Purdue would get something far more valuable: fuel for its public-relations machine.

SEVEN

Kiddie Dope

IT WAS A PROMOTION THAT GOT LAURA NAGEL HER FIRST real glimpse of the OxyContin crisis. Nagel had spent her career first working as an agent and then as a supervisor in the criminal division of the DEA, the high-profile part of the agency that goes after dealers and traffickers in illegal drugs such as heroin and cocaine. But in late 2000, she was promoted to head a little-known DEA section called the Office of Diversion Control; its job was to investigate cases where legal drugs such as OxyContin ended up on the street.

The promotion made Nagel one of the highest-ranking women at the DEA. She also was a person who did not waste time or shy away from a fight. Within weeks of taking her new job, she called together longtime staffers in the diversion unit to help her assess the OxyContin situation. Those officials had already reached a consensus. They believed that Purdue's claim that OxyContin might be less prone to abuse was wrong and had concluded the drugmaker wasn't doing enough to alert doctors and others about the problem. As a result, doctors were still prescribing the narcotic too freely, and it was winding up on the street. Nagel made a decision. With FDA officials seemingly unwilling to take on Purdue, the DEA would do so by going public about the havoc that OxyContin was causing. "It may take years to repair the damage that this drug has done," one DEA official said during a newspaper interview in early 2001.

Michael Friedman of Purdue quickly contacted Nagel, asking to meet. "We are writing as a consequence of the recent and widespread news reports concerning the illegal diversion and abuse in various areas of the country of one of this Company's analgesic products, OxyContin," Friedman wrote. He then added:

> We take this problem very seriously, as it is reminiscent of other events that have taken place over the years as new opioids have become available. The criminal element seems always able to devise means to evade the legal protective mechanisms that have been put in place and which are observed fully and conscientiously by the great bulk of licensed manufacturers, distributors and prescribers.
>
> Purdue Pharma has been working actively during the past year with federal, state and local officials to assist in their efforts for dealing with this drug diversion and abuse problem. We initiated a series of major programs to assure the OxyContin tablets are used in an appropriate and lawful manner. Purdue believes that these initiatives are important because OxyContin Tablets and other legal opioid-containing drugs are of critical importance for providing relief to numerous patients in moderate to severe pain.

Not long afterward, Friedman, David Haddox, and Howard Udell came to the DEA headquarters in Arlington, Virginia, to meet with Nagel. In a conference room on the building's sixth floor, Haddox turned on his laptop and started to make the company's standard presentation, which focused on the inadequate treatment of pain and the efforts by opioid advocates to use narcotics more aggressively. Nagel saw the presentation as a slickly produced dog-and-pony show and asked Haddox to shut off the computer so they could talk about the drug's abuse.

"This has gotten out of control," she said. "We need to do something."

She threw out ideas she had gotten from members of her staff. Given the growing number of drugstore robberies, it might be useful to restrict the dispensing of OxyContin to a limited number of drugstores in each town or city. Another suggestion was to limit prescribing privileges for OxyContin to doctors who were trained or certified in pain treatment. DEA officials such as Nagel had no direct control over how Purdue promoted its drugs—it was the FDA, not the DEA, that could change how Purdue marketed OxyContin by revising the drug's labeling language. Still, Nagel said she thought the company needed to curb the painkiller's wide availability, because it was an easy target for drug abusers and recreational users. Only Udell replied, saying, "We'll take that under advisement."

Nagel went on, telling the executives that she was greatly disturbed by newspaper accounts concerning overdose deaths as well as by reports that Purdue sales reps had pushed OxyContin too hard. Doctors were on the record saying that Purdue sales reps had tried to convince them to use OxyContin for insignificant injuries. A druggist was quoted as saying that a Purdue rep suggested a patient might sue him if he didn't fill OxyContin prescriptions. Friedman and Udell said the company was looking into the overdose reports but they denied any marketing excesses, emphasizing that they believed Purdue's sales policies to be extremely "conservative." They invited Nagel to alert them to any specific cases where a sales rep may have overstepped proper bounds, so they could investigate. After the Purdue team left the building, Nagel told one colleague that she felt the meeting had been a waste of time. The company hadn't agreed to do anything.

Ten days later, she received a five-page letter from Michael Friedman. Among other things, Friedman contended that the news media and critics of OxyContin had exaggerated the number of overdose deaths in which the drug might have played a role. He also claimed that published reports had inaccurately portrayed how Purdue had marketed the drug. He wrote:

> Purdue is working to gather information to help us understand the media reports of abuse, diversion and death attributed to OxyContin Tablets. As we discussed at the meeting, we do not want to minimize the significance of even one death; however, a clear understanding of the scope of the problem will help us all to better define how to deal with the problem. Prior to our meeting, we had received media reports of 59 deaths in Kentucky, 35 deaths in Maine, 20 deaths in Pennsylvania, and 28 deaths in Virginia. As you know, we are required to research all reported incidents of death and report our findings to FDA.
>
> This is what we know thus far:
>
> • We have obtained a letter from the State Medical Examiner's Office in Kentucky. This letter (March 1, 2001) states that "... I am unaware of any reliable data in Kentucky that proves that OxyContin is causing a lot of deaths. In the State M.E. Office, we are seeing an in-

crease in the number of deaths from ingesting several different prescription drugs and mixing them with alcohol. OxyContin is sometimes one of these drugs."

• We have obtained data from the Office of the Chief Medical Examiner in Maine. This data reports that during 1999 and part of 2000, there were 12 overdose deaths in which oxycodone was identified. Oxycodone was the sole chemical identified in only two cases, one of which was a suicide.

• As of this writing, we have only been able to obtain data from one county in Pennsylvania, Blair. . . . In this county, which encompasses Altoona, during the period from January 13, 1996 to December 1, 2000, there were 58 reported "Drug Deaths." Of these deaths, seven involved oxycodone as one of the agents causing death due to multiple drug toxicity. In no case was oxycodone listed as a single cause of death. We have no information at this point as to whether any of these deaths involved OxyContin.

• We are attempting to obtain data on the reported deaths in western Virginia involving oxycodone. We were told by one of the medical examiners in The Chief Medical Examiners Office of Virginia that there had been 31, not 28 deaths in western Virginia since 1997 involving oxycodone. Unfortunately, the authorities have not complied with our requests for information on the reported deaths. We have asked Attorney General Earley to help us obtain this information. At our meeting, you indicated that DEA might be able to obtain this information. We request that if you are able to do so, you consider sharing that information with us.

• As you can see, the facts that we have been able to obtain thus far are quite different than the media reports. We are not suggesting that there is no abuse and diversion. In fact, we know that such diversion and abuse exists. We just need to know how much, where and the source of diverted materials, so that we can all properly address the problem. As we discussed, we will send you summaries of our reports to the FDA on all of these cases. We would also appreciate any information that you can provide to us.

In concluding the letter, Friedman added that he believed much of the criticism about Purdue's marketing of OxyContin was coming from doctors who didn't believe that the use of strong opioids for moderate pain was acceptable practice. He rejected Nagel's suggestion of limiting the number of pharmacies dispensing OxyContin as impractical and added that it would create hardships for patients. Friedman acknowledged concerns that drug runners might be buying OxyContin at pharmacies in Mexico and smuggling it into the United States. As a result, he wrote, Purdue had decided to put special markings on tablets shipped to Mexico so that law-enforcement authorities would know that the pills came from there if they were seized during drug busts. The company had also modified its bonus plan for sales reps to encourage them to "sell to a broad base of doctors rather than focus on any single physician," his letter stated.

"I believe that we made great progress at our meeting in improving our understanding of this situation," Friedman concluded. "Purdue would like to continue to work with the DEA to stop the abuse and diversion of OxyContin and help address the broader problem of prescription drug abuse."

Nagel was infuriated by his response, which she viewed as Purdue's declaration that it was prepared to battle her on every point she'd raised. She also had no intention of backing down. "It's a screw-you letter," Nagel told one colleague.

The OxyContin crisis turned the DEA's view of drug abuse on its head. Illicit drugs had long been the agency's top priority, and criminal DEA agents referred derisively to prescription painkillers as "kiddie dope." But OxyContin made it clear that a legal drug could be just as devastating as any illicit substance. Not long after Nagel's meeting with the three Purdue executives, Florida officials announced that in 2001 there were more overdose deaths from OxyContin and other prescription painkillers than from heroin and cocaine.

The scope of the crisis involving legal drugs was unprecedented. But the DEA was ill-equipped to confront it. For years, investigators in the diversion division had played second fiddle to their criminal-division counterparts. They earned lower retirement benefits than criminal agents and weren't permitted to carry guns or conduct undercover operations. They also operated without the benefit of technological tools such as prescription-tracking data sold by IMS, the company once owned by the Sacklers. If DEA diversion investigators suspected a doctor of operating a pill mill, they couldn't push a button, as drugcompany sales reps could, to learn how frequently a physician was prescribing OxyContin and other opioids. Instead, they had to spend weeks traveling from pharmacy to pharmacy to compile that information by sorting through stacks of filled prescriptions that druggists were required to keep on file. Then, if they found adequate evidence to seize medical records from a doctor's office, they had to ask a DEA criminal agent to serve a search warrant, because they were not authorized to do so.

The division's staffing and morale problems could be traced back to 1994 and the appointment of Thomas Constantine as DEA administrator. During his five-year tenure, Constantine, a former New York State Police Department superintendent, gained a reputation as a polarizing figure and was disliked by field agents within both the diversion and criminal divisions. But while Constantine doubled the number of staffers on the DEA's criminal side, he saw those involved in its prescription-drug operation as meddlesome regulators.

Constantine told a group of drug-company executives that he understood their impatience with regulators, because he had experienced similar frustrations with workplace-safety officials while heading the New York State police. They "used to come into my barracks and check to see if the shoe polish was edible," Constantine said. When one official within DEA's diversion division confronted him about the unit's stepchild treatment, he spelled out his bottom line. "Has a diversion investigator ever been killed in the line of duty?" he asked. The conversation ended when he was told that none had.

Opioid advocates also treated the DEA diversion division as a favored whipping boy, depicting its agents the way gun lovers portrayed firearms agents—as jackbooted government thugs who ripped prescription pads out of the hands of well-meaning doctors. The medical profession's sudden acceptance of opioids made diversion agents almost seem superfluous, and by the mid-1990s the unit had all but given up investigating doctors for illegally prescribing narcotics.

In taking over the division, Nagel, who was tall and thin with a narrow face and dirty-blond hair, was confronted with not only a public health crisis involving OxyContin but also a dispirited,

alienated staff. Nagel viewed OxyContin as the forerunner of a
new generation of high-powered painkillers already in the pharmaceutical industry's pipeline, medications that, sold without
added safeguards from the FDA, would unleash even more public chaos. In 1999, Purdue executives had publicly announced
plans to market a time-release version of the narcotic hydromorphone, the powerful and addicting drug that had earned the
nickname "drugstore heroin" when first sold in the 1920s as Dilaudid. Purdue was already selling the drug in Canada, but the
FDA found problems with Purdue's application and had delayed
its approval in the United States.

For all of her opposition to OxyContin's marketing and distribution, Nagel was against recalling the drug. For one thing, she
thought that federal officials did not have sufficient legal grounds
to do so. In addition, she believed that the threat posed by the
painkiller could be sharply reduced if Purdue stepped back from
promoting it for the treatment of patients with "moderate" pain,
which accounted for much of the drug's use. Because it was clear
Purdue had no intention of doing this, she decided to use another forum to put pressure on the company—the court of public opinion.

In May 2001, the DEA announced the start of a sweeping
program to reduce the abuse of OxyContin. Agency officials said
it was the first time they had targeted a specific brand-name prescription drug, rather than a class of medications, for special
attention.

Nagel knew that she could be hotheaded—even volatile at
times—so she assigned one of her top aides, Terrance Woodworth, a longtime diversion-division official, to be her public
voice. Woodworth began to give media interviews challenging
Purdue to restrict its marketing effort and drop its contention

that OxyContin was less likely to be abused than similar narcotics.

Woodworth, who was known as Terry, told one newspaper that DEA officials believed that Purdue's aggressive promotion of OxyContin was causing physicians to try it before other drugs. "The DEA is extremely concerned that many doctors are prescribing this strong narcotic as an initial treatment for many types of pain," Woodworth said.

He also squared off against David Haddox on television talk shows. OxyContin's abuse had "skyrocketed in various communities, from Maine to Florida, all along the East Coast," Woodworth said on one program. "And it's moving into the central United States. We're getting reports from Arizona and Nevada, Washington and Oregon, and even Alaska is reporting a growing abuse problem."

In response, Haddox maintained the company's stance that there had been some instances of abuse but insisted that the focus needed to remain on pain patients and their needs. "I think that one of the nice things about medicine in this country is that doctors have a lot of choices," he replied. "And what you've heard thus far this morning on the segment is the problems with abuse of the drug. No one's talked about the patients. There are fifty million patients in this country who have chronic pain that's not being managed appropriately every single day. OxyContin is one of the choices that doctors have available to them to treat that."

Nagel's campaign was not just aimed at Purdue. She also hoped to goad officials at the FDA into action. The mission of the FDA—which approves the use of beneficial drugs—and that of the DEA—which makes sure such medications don't fall into the wrong hands—are meant to complement each other. But in trying to wrestle with OxyContin, those separate mandates came into conflict and set off a decade of governmental paralysis that would instead widen the scope of the opioid crisis.

Purdue began its own campaign against Nagel, telling reporters that the DEA was beating up on the company to enhance its own prestige. Nagel's colleagues at the Justice Department, which oversees the DEA, alerted her that Purdue executives, in an effort to make an end run around her, had used a political lobbyist to arrange a meeting with her superiors. They invited her to the meeting but didn't tell Purdue she would be there. When Michael Friedman and Howard Udell walked into a Justice Department conference room, they were surprised to see Nagel. "We were going to stop in and see you while we were in town," Udell managed to say.

Also at the meeting was Purdue president Richard Sackler. Like his father and uncles, Richard, who was fifty-six in 2001, had trained as a physician before entering the drug business. He was known around Purdue headquarters as a pleasant person, though he appeared ill at ease in groups; while he addressed the company's sales force once a year, he rarely stayed afterward to mingle. Those who did business with Purdue were left with the strong impression that Raymond and Mortimer Sackler made the big decisions. But Richard's presence signified the gravity of this meeting nonetheless. As Sackler took his seat in the conference room, Laura Nagel passed him her business card, and he lined it up on the table's edge alongside the other cards he had received.

When the meeting began, Purdue's executives assured Justice Department officials that they had promoted OxyContin responsibly and now were doing everything possible to curb its abuse. Sackler, who was dressed casually in a tweed sports jacket and a shirt with a button-down collar, didn't speak much. Then he broke into the company's formal presentation to remark that OxyContin was an extremely good drug.

Nagel leaned across the table, bringing her face close to his. "People are dying, do you understand that?" she told him. "And I'm not going to back down."

Sackler looked shaken and stared down at the business cards in front of him. "I think I understand that," he replied.

After the meeting, however, it was Purdue that went on the attack, against both the DEA and Nagel. In June 2001, Howard Udell wrote Nagel to notify her that *USA Today* was about to publish an editorial about OxyContin. His letter included the text of an email message written by an official from Purdue's public-relations department who had dealt with the newspaper.

"USA Today is planning an editorial on how DEA is handling the OxyContin abuse and diversion issue," the Purdue PR official had written. "It will probably appear on Wednesday of this week. Based on conversations that I and David Haddox had with the writer, it appears that the piece will be critical of the DEA's actions. Both David and I took pain to avoid taking an adversarial position to the DEA."

The tone of the *USA Today* editorial was clear from its headline, DEA OVERREACHES IN EFFORT TO STOP ABUSE OF PAINKILLER. It stated that the agency's proposals to restrict to pain specialists the doctors prescribing OxyContin would harm patients because there were only four thousand such specialists in the country. It also argued that the DEA's singular focus on OxyContin's role was misguided because it ignored the fact that forty other prescription drugs contained oxycodone as their active ingredient.

"More importantly, there's little evidence that restricting patients' access to painkillers will do much to fight drug abuse," the *USA Today* editorial stated. "Only last year, The Journal of the American Medical Association published a study, based in part on the DEA's own data, concluding that increased prescribing of powerful painkillers did not increase drug abuse."

David Haddox had pointed reporters toward that same 2000 *JAMA* study since the public controversy over OxyContin began. But Purdue executives and their allies misrepresented that study much as they had the three early reports they used to argue for the safety of opioids.

The *JAMA* study at issue was based on data gathered through a government-run system known as the Drug Abuse Warning Network, or DAWN for short, which collects reports of hospital emergency-room admissions for prescription-drug overdoses. But the DAWN data on which the report in *JAMA* was based had been collected between 1990 and 1996, a period that predated OxyContin's appearance. In addition, the study's lead author was a well-known opioid advocate, David Joranson, the researcher at the University of Wisconsin whose think tank had received millions of dollars from Purdue and other pharmaceutical companies. In a press release that accompanied the study's publication in 2000, Joranson and his colleagues celebrated the data as fulfilling their prophecy that the wider medical use of narcotics wouldn't lead to increased abuse. "This study suggests that increased use of opioid pain medications resulting in abuse may be based more on myth than reality," one of Joranson's coauthors wrote.

But that illusory claim had been dispelled even before Joranson's study appeared. Beginning in 1998, two years after the cutoff date of his study, the number of emergency-room reports involving prescription narcotics started to soar. Between 1994 and 2001, DAWN data showed, references in emergency-room reports to oxycodone-containing painkillers such as OxyContin climbed by 350 percent. This rate of growth far outpaced the rise in incidents involving hydrocodone-containing painkillers like

Vicodin, even though those drugs were prescribed three times more often. In fact, by 2001 the total number of reports mentioning oxycodone-containing painkillers was fast approaching those for hydrocodone-based drugs. It was a tragic marker of Purdue's success in marketing OxyContin.

The company, hoping to forestall any significant actions against the drug, sent a memo in late 2000 to its sales reps, stating that it was "vital" for them to be forthright about the drug's abuse. Purdue also tinkered with OxyContin's labeling claim that its time-release formulation might lower its appeal to abusers by adding that the claim applied when the drug was "used properly for the management of pain."

In April 2001, FDA officials and Purdue executives finally had their first face-to-face meeting to discuss ways to deal with the painkiller's misuse. Agency officials agreed with Purdue that pain patients, with very rare exceptions, saw only benefits from OxyContin, an assumption that in later years would prove deeply flawed. But FDA officials opened the meeting by recommending significant changes to the types of claims Purdue would be allowed to make for OxyContin. One area involved changes to the medical conditions—or "indications," in FDA jargon—for which the painkiller's use was recommended. The other area involved the drug's warning label.

According to the minutes of the meeting, a medical reviewer for the FDA stated:

> The indication of "moderate to severe pain for patients who need to be on opiates for more than a few days" is broad and may not adequately reflect the intended population. The label should clearly state that this drug should be used only by patients who require opiates for an extended period of time, that it should not be utilized

for first-time treatment of pain, and that it is not for
intermittent use.

The reviewer, Sharon Hertz, further stated that a "black-box
warning," the most severe warning the FDA can apply to a
medication, might be appropriate for OxyContin. Dr. Cynthia G.
McCormick, the director of the agency's division of anesthetics,
critical care, and addiction drug products, questioned the value
of some of the scientific studies provided to the FDA to evaluate
OxyContin. Still another official remarked that he believed Oxy-
Contin's label "will need a major overhaul."

The Purdue executives at the FDA meeting said they wanted
to cooperate with the agency. But it's clear in the FDA report that
they were concerned that any actions directed specifically at
OxyContin would, in their view, unfairly stigmatize the drug.

> Purdue said they are having a difficult time understand-
> ing how abuse of OxyContin differs from abuse of other
> Schedule II drugs. They are concerned that they may
> create a perception that this drug is different. They
> would like to concur with the Agency's requests if the
> Agency will request the same of other companies.

FDA officials responded that there were issues unique to Oxy-
Contin that needed to be addressed. Doctors mistakenly believed
that the drug wasn't as powerful as morphine and, as a result,
they were using it for "frivolous" purposes such as the treatment
of dental pain. When the meeting ended, an FDA official asked if
the Purdue executives had accurate data about the number and
types of patients using OxyContin. They claimed that the only
data the company had was "anecdotal."

In July 2001, four months after the negotiations between the

FDA and Purdue began, the company announced a series of voluntary changes to OxyContin's labeling. Purdue would drop the claim that OxyContin's time-release formulation might reduce its risk of abuse compared to traditional painkillers. Instead, the new label would read, "Oxycodone can be abused in a manner similar to other opioid agonists, legal or illicit." Purdue also agreed to put a black-box warning on OxyContin and use language to indicate that it should be used to treat extended or chronic pain rather than incidents lasting "a few days or more." The company announced a plan to better detect OxyContin's abuse as well, by collecting relevant reports from drug-treatment centers.

Years later, one top FDA official admitted that the agency response to Purdue was an acknowledgment that it had blundered in approving claims for OxyContin in 1995.

"It clearly was being perceived as a severe problem when young, otherwise healthy people are dying and communities are having their people decimated," that official said. "We began to become acutely aware of how inaccurate the original label was and how it had probably contributed to the problem."

Purdue sent out an alert about the new warning and prescription information by overnight mail to 800,000 doctors and pharmacists nationwide. In that letter, the company noted that it was "proud to be the first pharmaceutical manufacturer to voluntarily revise prescribing information" for a tightly controlled narcotic that addressed its abuse and diversion.

By then, Laura Nagel was preparing to send out her own letter. Unlike Purdue and officials at the FDA, she didn't believe that the danger posed by OxyContin was limited to drug abusers. She also told colleagues that nothing incensed her more than Purdue's apparent refusal to acknowledge its drug's role in overdose deaths. Nagel had a fantasy in which she forced Purdue executives to watch a slide show depicting every person who had died of an OxyContin-related overdose, along with a narration of a life tragically cut short. The drug company's executives would hear about the college student who had died of an overdose the first time he tried OxyContin at a party; they would see a picture of a young teenage girl who had fatally overdosed; and so on.

Nagel knew from her experiences as a criminal agent that society could accept a certain number of drug-overdose deaths per year. Few tears were spilled over dead junkies. But she had come to believe that OxyContin's toll was unacceptable. The company was free to dispute the drug's role in every one of those deaths. It would be legal suicide for Purdue to take any other position, but Nagel was determined to tally the deaths as best she could and try to understand whether pain patients were among them.

In mid-2001, the DEA sent letters to medical examiners and coroners in more than thirty states, asking them for specific information. The agency wanted every medical examiner's report, autopsy report, and police report connected with any drug-overdose death during the previous eighteen months in which oxycodone had turned up in the blood or bodily fluids of the dead.

About that same time, OxyContin had attracted the attention of other federal officials. One of them was an investigator named Gregory Wood, who was based in the United States Attorney's office in Roanoke, Virginia, and worked on cases involving fraud against government healthcare programs such as Medicare and Medicaid. Along with other cops and federal agents in western Virginia, he had watched the parallel growth of OxyContin and crime.

Like Nagel and Art Van Zee, Wood tended toward the obsessive. In February 2001, he sent out the first edition of a digital news digest he created that contained every media account he could find mentioning OxyContin and crimes connected to it. Those regular emails, which were known to readers as the *Wood Reports*, became a chronicle of the catastrophe's course, and Wood encouraged recipients to share them. "Updates are not restricted to law enforcement," a header on each email stated.

Wood also spent lots of time in places like Lee County, investigating doctors suspected of running pill mills. During his travels, he talked to druggists who recounted how Purdue sales reps had repeatedly claimed that OxyContin was safer than competing painkillers or that it couldn't be abused. Wood was aware that sales reps invariably hyped the drugs they sold. But he also knew a lot about FDA regulations, including those that made it illegal for a company to make unapproved claims for a medication. The arrests of prescribing doctors and the pharmacy break-ins cited in his news digest, Wood and other investigators began to suspect, were symptoms of a far more significant crime, one that lay inside Purdue Pharma.

EIGHT

Purple Peelers

BY MID-2001, FEDERAL LAWMAKERS ALSO STARTED TO WONder when Purdue executives had first learned about the abuse of OxyContin and whether they could have done more to curb it. And that August, a panel of the House of Representatives Energy and Commerce Committee held a public hearing at a meeting hall in Bensalem, Pennsylvania, a working-class suburb of Philadelphia. Here, company officials would offer their first testimony about those questions under oath.

Lawmakers had chosen Bensalem as the site for the hearing because an area doctor, Richard Paolino, had been recently arrested on charges of running a pill mill that had spewed out thousands of prescriptions for OxyContin. Over a five-month period, Paolino—who was an osteopath, not a cancer specialist or a pain expert—had written 1,200 prescriptions for OxyContin, or about nine prescriptions a day. During Paolino's time prescribing, five people around Bensalem, four of them teenagers, died of drug overdoses involving oxycodone.

The hearing took place at a pivotal time for Purdue. Only a month had passed since the company, following discussions with the FDA, had sent out its nationwide alert warning doctors about OxyContin abuse. Some states, concerned that the costly painkiller was consuming their budget for prescription drugs, had begun to require doctors to obtain special approval before prescribing it. The drug was still a blockbuster, bringing in more than $1 billion in sales, but the controversies surrounding it had slowed its rate of anticipated growth.

Along with Michael Friedman and Howard Udell, the group of company officials at the hearing included Dr. Paul Goldenheim, Purdue's top medical officer, and its chief public-relations official, Robin Hogen.

In his opening statement to the congressional panel, Friedman tackled the central issue first. He said Purdue had first become aware of the abuse of OxyContin in early 2000, as a result of articles in Maine newspapers and when the U.S. Attorney there sent out an alert to doctors in the state.

"Purdue immediately implemented a response team that included some of the company's top executives and scientists, including those who are here today," Friedman said. "That team has committed Purdue to an unprecedented program to combat abuse and diversion."

The congressman leading the panel, Representative James C. Greenwood of Pennsylvania, did not ask Friedman why Purdue had relied on newspaper articles to monitor abuse of its drug. Instead, he focused on the more fundamental issue of the IMS database that showed how doctors were prescribing OxyContin. If Purdue had real-time data from the IMS database, he asked, why weren't company officials alarmed when they saw how many prescriptions Dr. Paolino was writing?

"When you see a doctor who is not associated with Fox Chase Cancer Center but is a little osteopath here in Bensalem, doing this vast number [of OxyContin prescriptions], what do you do with that information?" Greenwood asked Friedman.

Friedman's response seemed well rehearsed. "We have learned over the years that the absolute number of prescriptions that a physician is prescribing is, in and of itself, not an indicator of the doctor doing something wrong. We don't measure or assess how well a doctor practices medicine. We are not in the office with a physician and a patient, observing the examination or involved in that process. We know, for example—"

Greenwood cut him off. "Why do you want that information, then?" he asked.

"Well, we use that information to understand what is happening in terms of the development of use of our product in any area," Friedman replied.

"You want to see how successful your marketing techniques are?" Greenwood asked.

"Sure," said Friedman, glancing back at his Purdue colleagues for support.

Greenwood then returned to his first question and asked Friedman to explain why Purdue used IMS data to measure its marketing success but not to monitor whether doctors were properly prescribing OxyContin.

"That is the other side of your responsibility," Greenwood said. "Why wouldn't you have been using this data to make sure that the Dr. Paolinos of the world weren't wrecking the reputation of your product?"

Howard Udell leaned forward and whispered to Friedman.

"I think Mr. Udell might be able to respond to that more," Friedman said, yielding the witness table to the lawyer.

When he took over, Udell insisted that Purdue couldn't have known from the IMS data alone that Paolino was running a pill mill. Law-enforcement officials, he said, were far better suited than a drugmaker like Purdue to investigate problem doctors.

His answer didn't satisfy Greenwood. "It seems to me that

your company has a responsibility to be looking at this data and not relying on what law enforcement tells you," he said. "I don't understand why that hasn't been something that you have been aggressively doing."

Udell decided little was to be gained from arguing. "I think we learned a lot from the case of Dr. Paolino," he responded. "The picture that is painted in the newspaper is of a horrible, bad actor, someone who preyed on this community, who caused untold suffering. And he fooled us all. He fooled law enforcement. He fooled the DEA. He fooled local law enforcement. He fooled us." Udell's quick thinking managed to blunt Greenwood's questions, and the Bensalem hearing ended without any damage to Purdue's reputation.

Company officials set out clear lines of defense at the hearing that they would repeatedly invoke in the face of other lawmakers' and investigators' questions. The first defense was that the company couldn't have known if some doctors were "bad actors" who peddled pills, because it wasn't in a position to judge how doctors practiced. But more crucially, Purdue executives would persistently claim, both in sworn testimony before Congress and also in letters sent to the company's sales reps, that there had been a defining moment when Purdue had become aware that OxyContin was being abused. The precise time would vary by a few weeks, but executives insisted that the company only became aware of the problem in the early months of 2000, when Jay McCloskey, the U.S. Attorney in Maine, issued his alert.

In December 2001, four months after the Bensalem hearing, Paul Goldenheim testified before a Senate panel that reports of OxyContin's abuse had taken Purdue entirely by surprise, because the company had not seen any "unusual" abuse or diversion of OxyContin's predecessor, MS Contin, during the seventeen years that powerful opioid had been on the market. "Purdue had no reason to expect otherwise with OxyContin," Goldenheim said.

But the bright lines that Purdue officials sought to draw, federal investigators later discovered, weren't clear-cut. In fact, three years before Goldenheim's testimony, Purdue executives learned that MS Contin had become a favored street drug and that OxyContin might face a similar fate. That information came from a study performed by researchers from the University of British Columbia in Vancouver that was published in 1998 in the prestigious *Canadian Medical Association Journal*.

The university researchers hadn't set out to look for MS Contin abuse. Instead, they decided to interview drug abusers and dealers in a seedy downtown section of Vancouver to learn about the types of prescription drugs for sale there and the prices those drugs were commanding. The prevailing wisdom, as Purdue had told the FDA when seeking approval for OxyContin's special claim, was that the time-release opioids such as MS Contin and OxyContin would be less appealing to drug abusers. But to their surprise, the Canadian researchers found that MS Contin was turning up frequently on the street for sale and also had the highest black-market price of any prescription narcotic, because of its high levels of pure morphine.

Drug users had also learned how to defeat MS Contin's time-release system by scraping off a tablet's outer coating and then crushing and dissolving the pill so that the morphine within it could be injected, researchers reported. MS Contin tablets had been nicknamed "peelers"—because you peeled away a tablet's outer coating. A green MS Contin tablet, which contained 15 milligrams of morphine, was called a "green peeler." A stronger, purple-colored tablet containing 30 milligrams was known as a "purple peeler."

That same issue of the *Canadian Medical Association Journal* contained an editorial written by an emergency-room physician, Dr. Brian Goldman, which warned that OxyContin could also end up on the street. In the editorial, he said the results of the Vancouver study contradicted safety claims—made by Purdue and others—for time-release narcotics. Goldman wrote that the Vancouver researchers

> appear to be among the first to publish evidence on the street value of controlled-release opioid preparations (so-called "peelers"). It has been argued previously that controlled-release preparations might be less desirable as drugs of abuse than immediate-release pharmaceuticals. The relatively high street price of controlled-release opioid analgesics reported in this study clearly indicates that these drugs are coveted. This should ring alarm bells. The manufacturer of one brand of morphine sulfate tablets (MS Contin) has warned that injection of the drug obtained by street crude methods could result in local tissue necrosis and pulmonary granuloma [conditions produced by the injection of talc, which is used as a binding agent in the manufacture of pharmaceutical tablets]. These issues need to be resolved.

Then Goldman referred directly to the risk posed by OxyContin: "Now that controlled-release oxycodone [OxyContin] has been licensed in Canada, we can expect that it and other controlled-release opioid analgesics will also find their way onto the black market."

There is no evidence that Purdue sent the Canadian report to the FDA or to doctors in the United States. The drugmaker apparently had good reasons not to—if widely publicized, the study and editorial would have undermined the foundation of the high-powered marketing campaign that Purdue had just launched for OxyContin. Years later, Brian Goldman, who was a consultant to Purdue at the time his editorial was published, would say that the company never contacted him about it.

By 1999, a year before the Maine warning, Purdue officials were made aware of OxyContin abuse by another source—the company's own sales reps. And one of those reps, Kimberly Keith, promoted OxyContin to doctors in Lee County, including Art Van Zee.

Keith, after each visit to a physician in her territory, wrote a "call report," a brief memo describing that meeting. Such memos were a standard practice in the drug industry, and a rep used them to make note of any issues that a doctor might have brought up about a drug and to jot down ideas about ways to increase the doctor's prescribing.

One doctor Keith regularly visited was Richard Norton, who practiced in Duffield, Virginia, just twenty miles east of Van Zee's clinic in St. Charles. And by mid-1999, she was filing call reports about how Norton's patients were abusing OxyContin by crushing a tablet with their teeth and then swallowing or snorting oxycodone. (Her notes, written quickly, contained abbreviations, typos, and misspellings.)

After one of these visits to Norton, she wrote:

> SAID PATS [patients] NOT DOING SO WELL BCAUSE CHEWING OXY ETC, UPSET THAT CAN BREAK TABLET DOWN [.] NOT THAT THEY HAVE FIGURED OUT HOW TO DO IT. DISUCSSED GIVING IT TO THE RIGHT PATIENTS WOULDN'T BE A CONCERN.

Two weeks later, Keith filed a new call report, reflecting Norton's comments made during another visit with him. It read:

SAID VERY DISAPPOINTED THAT PURDUE DOESN'T
MAKE A CHEMICAL DELIVERY VS A MECHANICAL.
ASKED WHY, BCAUSE PATS ARE CHEWING OXY-
CONTIN AND GETTING A RUSH. NOT SEEING LOT
OF PATIENTS WITH NECROSIS [from hypodermic in-
jection]. SAID WAS GOING TO MS CONTIN BCAUSE
DIDN'T SEEM TO GET THE BUZZ OR EURPHOIA
LIKE WITH OXYCONTIN, NEED TO DISCUSS NEXT
TIME.

Purdue also became aware in 1999 of increasing newspaper
articles about OxyContin's abuse as well as the arrests of doctors
prescribing it. Early that year, for example, police and state drug
agents stormed a pain clinic located in a small rural town in
northern California called Redding. They arrested the clinic's
operator, Dr. Frank Fisher, who had written hundreds of prescriptions for OxyContin, and charged him with fraud as well as
murder in connection with the deaths of three of his patients
from drug overdoses that involved oxycodone. Prosecutors
showed that in 1998 Fisher had written a startling 46 percent of
all the prescriptions for OxyContin issued through a California
state program for low-income patients. That same year, a pharmacy near his office had purchased nearly four times as much
OxyContin and other oxycodone-containing painkillers as any
other retail drugstore in the United States. The drugstore's owners denied any wrongdoing, while Fisher maintained that his
prescribing practices reflected new medical views about the
need to use such drugs more aggressively in pain treatment.

Court records show that expert witnesses working for the
state of California contacted Purdue in 1999 for information
about OxyContin because the drug was still a relatively new
product on the market. Years later, Fisher's defense lawyers

would recount that they also had quickly got in touch with Purdue to seek the company's assistance in mounting his defense. Fisher later said he spoke directly to a Purdue physician as well, who told him that the company would not get involved in his case, because its executives were conservative and liked to avoid controversy.

By then Purdue was monitoring media reports for any mention of OxyContin abuse. That spring two Purdue sales reps turned up at the offices of a tiny newspaper in West Virginia, *The Weirton Daily Times*, to ask for a copy of a recently published article in which William Beatty, the head of a local narcotics task force, warned that a new drug scourge was taking hold in the area. "Too much heroin and too many Oxycontins are hitting the streets in the Upper Ohio Valley," Beatty's article said. At about that same time, a Purdue sales rep in western Pennsylvania reported back to the company that authorities there had sent out an alert to area doctors about both MS Contin and OxyContin. The drugs "have found a niche in the illegal recreational drug use setting," the alert stated. "Pharmaceutical drug abusers have found a way to circumvent the oral administration to negate the long-lasting effect of the drugs, thus producing a 'speed' type of high from the drugs. The local street price runs from $30–$60 per pill."

Before 1999 ended, Purdue would learn about the arrest of other doctors on OxyContin-related charges. One of those cases involved a Florida doctor, James F. Graves, who was charged with manslaughter in connection with the overdose deaths of four patients to whom he had prescribed a combination of drugs. Graves, a former Navy doctor, had bounced from job to job before finally opening an office in Pace, Florida, a small town near the city of Pensacola in the state's panhandle section. He didn't have any special training in treating pain, but his small office was attracting large numbers of patients complaining of pain. He prescribed them a mix of medications dubbed by local pharmacists the "Graves cocktail." It included narcotic pain-killers such as OxyContin and Lortab as well as a tranquilizer, Xanax.

His patients who died all had histories of drug abuse, but some of their parents would later testify at Graves's trial that they had pleaded with him not to prescribe their children more drugs. "Word spread that he was the go-to doctor," a Florida prosecutor told a jury during the physician's trial. "He's no different than a drug dealer."

A Purdue sales rep, Leon V. Dulion, testified that he started hearing complaints in 1999 from area pharmacists that Graves was inappropriately prescribing OxyContin, particularly higher-strength tablets that contained 40 or 80 milligrams of oxyco-done. He was also concerned that Graves was using a Purdue promotional campaign to give patients free samples of OxyContin.

Within the pharmaceutical industry, it is standard practice for sales reps to drop off small free-sample packets of a new drug at doctors' offices as a way to encourage physicians to prescribe the medication to patients. Under DEA rules, drug companies are not permitted to give out free samples of narcotics, but Purdue and other opioid manufacturers had found a work-around. Instead of sample packets, Purdue sales reps annually distributed thousands of coupons to doctors, each one good for either a seven-day or a thirty-day trial supply of OxyContin. A physician could give a patient a coupon to take to the drugstore and get the painkiller for free. In internal budgets, Purdue put the annual cost of its giveaway program at $4 million.

Dulion told prosecutors that in the first few months of 1999 he received thirty such coupons and gave six of them to Graves.

Each one was good for a free thirty-day supply of the painkiller, a quantity large enough for a patient to develop significant dependence or even addiction to an opioid. Then Dulion overheard a conversation in another doctor's office that suggested to him that Graves was using the OxyContin coupons to make money. Two people waiting to see the physician were discussing the types of drugs available for sale on the street; their conversation turned to Graves and how he used to give out a coupon "that would get you all your OxyContin for free" if the patient agreed to sign up for a long-distance telephone service that he was marketing as a side business. Dulion also testified that the same two people discussed the popularity of OxyContin with drug abusers. One of them said, "On the street the number-one abused drug is crack cocaine, which they call the devil's dick, followed by Oxy-Contin, which they refer to as the devil's balls."

In mid-1999, Frank Fisher, the California doctor, was released from jail after the murder charges against him were reduced to manslaughter. (All felony charges against him were later dropped, and he was acquitted of related misdemeanor charges after a trial in 2004.) Fisher remained a strong believer in Oxy-Contin's value and, not long after his release, he attended a pain-management presentation sponsored by Purdue.

Years later, he would recall that he was stunned to hear the Purdue speaker repeatedly insist that the painkiller couldn't be abused, because of its time-release packaging. "All the nurses there were laughing about it," Fisher said. He was so upset by the incident, he said, that he phoned Purdue's headquarters, where his call was directed to David Haddox, who had then just started working for the drug company. Fisher said he recounted the speaker's remarks. "David, you know that what your lecturers are telling people isn't true," he recalled saying.

Fisher described Haddox as sounding very concerned during

their phone call, adding that the Purdue official had asked for the speaker's name. Fisher never learned how, or even if, his complaint was addressed. He never heard back from Haddox.

Haddox would later downplay early reports about OxyContin's abuse, describing them as "dribs and drabs." But that was not the case. In time, new evidence would emerge to show that in late 1999—long before Purdue executives testified in Congress—Haddox had urged them to enact a crisis-response plan to OxyContin's growing abuse. His call went unheeded.

NINE

The Body Count

As 2002 BEGAN, PURDUE WAS A COMPANY IN CRISIS. IT FACED investigations from federal officials such as Laura Nagel as well as inquiries from state officials. Scrutiny of the company by the news media remained intense, and plaintiffs' lawyers had started to file a growing number of lawsuits against it on behalf of people who said they had become addicted to OxyContin.

The controversy engulfing the company was unlike anything it had experienced during its fifty-year history. But as 2002 unfolded, Purdue began to turn the tide by relying on the kinds of tools and tactics that the Sackler brothers had long deployed: The company used money, job offers, and other favors to coopt, influence, or defeat its critics or potential opponents.

Among the first to climb on Purdue's bandwagon was the U.S. Attorney in Maine, Jay McCloskey, who had been the first federal official to alert doctors about the hazards of OxyContin. McCloskey began doing legal work for Purdue in May of 2001, immediately after he stepped down as prosecutor. In fact, there's evidence that he and Purdue were in contact about future work while he was still in public office. An internal Purdue memo written in March 2001 showed a rundown of efforts the com-

pany was then undertaking to deal with the OxyContin controversy, including scheduled meetings with public officials. It read:

> a) AG [Maine's state attorney general] wants to
> take over our relationship [as the point person on the
> OxyContin issue] now that McCloskey is leaving. RH
> [Robin Hogen, head of Purdue public relations] to call
> and schedule a meeting.

> b) We will try to schedule a follow-up with McCloskey
> while we are there; he called looking for business for
> his new law practice.

> c) News release put out on $3/8$ on tamper-resistant
> prescription pad program; McCloskey prepped to field
> questions and compliment PPLP [Purdue Pharma] for
> our initiative in "doing the right thing."

Years later, McCloskey vehemently disputed any suggestion
that he had contacted the company seeking work prior to leaving his job as U.S. Attorney. But he was hardly the only former
public official to end up on Purdue's payroll. The company soon
hired a number of former DEA agents as well as local law-
enforcement officials from Virginia and other states hit hard by
OxyContin abuse. It also poured money into organizations representing local and federal drug agents, including the National
Association of Drug Diversion Investigators. At the group's annual meeting in 2001, Purdue's David Haddox showed attendees
slides of newspaper reports, which he contended overstated the
scope of the OxyContin problem and the drug's addictive potential. One attendee passed a note to a colleague that read: "This is
like Philip Morris saying that cigarettes don't cause cancer."
Professional organizations, whether they represent doctors or

cops, like to believe that corporate contributions have no effect on their policies or public positions. But groups that happily took Purdue's money to underwrite their annual conferences or pay for steak dinners never seemed to realize how deeply those funds could corrode an institution's mission.

At its 2000 meeting, a group that represents state-level drug regulators, the National Association of State Controlled Substances Authorities (NASCSA), heard an urgent call to action about a looming opioid crisis. A New York State official, John Eadie, told his colleagues that federal data showed that young people were increasingly experimenting with legal opioids and that a failure to act would create a new generation of drug abusers as well as a legal backlash against prescription narcotics that would imperil the needs of pain patients. If the situation was "not reversed quickly," Eadie warned, there was a high risk of injuring "a very significant number of children and young adults through accidents, addiction, overdoses, and death."

But two years later, members of NASCSA, which took money from Purdue, heard a very different message at their conference, one about corporate spin and image-making rather than public health. The guest speaker that year was a "crisis management" expert hired by Purdue, Eric Dezenhall, who entertained safety regulators with a talk entitled "Who Survives the Media and Why."

By 2002, Art Van Zee's attempts to warn the public about Oxy-Contin had floundered. The citizens' petition he had launched at Lee High asking the FDA to recall the drug had attracted little attention outside Lee County and had garnered only 8,500 signatures. Meanwhile, the Internet site that he had created to publicize the recall effort had received plenty of negative messages. "Are you a real doctor?" one person emailed him. "If you are, you should not be. I wouldn't send my dog to be treated by you."

Lawmakers also gave him a chilly reception when he testified in February 2002 before a Senate panel. During the long drive he made with Sue Ella from western Virginia to the nation's capital, Van Zee had rehearsed what he planned to say. "What are the most important points I can make?" he asked her again and again. "I only have five minutes. What are the three most important points I should make?"

He entered the Senate hearing room wearing his only suit and a colorful Jerry Garcia necktie from his mother. Several Purdue executives, including Dr. Paul Goldenheim, who was also set to testify, were already there. Van Zee spoke first, bluntly telling the panel that Purdue should be required to recall OxyContin and reformulate it to be resistant to abuse.

"First," he said, "there has been an obvious problem with physicians misprescribing and overprescribing this drug. Secondly, this epidemic has been a vicious indicator of the alarming degree of prescription-drug abuse in this society. Thirdly, and perhaps . . . closest to this committee and the FDA is that the promotion and marketing of OxyContin by Purdue Pharma has played a major role in this problem."

Members of the Senate panel quickly made it clear to Van Zee that they had no intention of doing more than they already were to curb the drug. But it was Senator Christopher Dodd of Connecticut, Purdue's home state, who began to aggressively question Van Zee, challenging him to provide evidence to prove that Purdue's promotion of OxyContin had spurred the drug's abuse. He also pointed out that areas like Lee County had had problems with prescription painkillers long before OxyContin's arrival.

Dodd's comments mirrored the talking points Purdue executives had been making to defend OxyContin and their marketing methods. That was hardly surprising, because the Connecticut Democrat had met with Howard Udell and other Purdue officials weeks before the hearing took place. In a follow-up letter to Dodd, Udell wrote that Purdue had "no reason to expect" Oxy-Contin would be abused, because the company had been un-aware of any significant abuse of its predecessor drug, MS Contin.

In response to Dodd's question, Van Zee replied that while he didn't have data to prove his point, it was common sense to assume that when a drug company aggressively promoted a narcotic in areas known for drug abuse, it was a "recipe for commercial success and public-health problems." Later in 2002, Senator Dodd received $10,000 in campaign contributions from Purdue's political-action committee, ten times more than it gave to any other lawmaker that year.

Purdue's success in quelling congressional opposition was replicated in the courtroom. To defend itself against the growing number of OxyContin-related lawsuits, the company had hired two of the biggest law firms in the United States, King & Spalding and Chadbourne & Parke. Both firms were formidable, with a depth of legal talent and experience.

In squaring off against Purdue, plaintiffs' lawyers faced an-other problem—their own clients. Most lawsuit claimants had abused other drugs prior to OxyContin, making it virtually im-possible for lawyers to show that Purdue was responsible for their addiction. Lawsuits against the company were routinely dismissed and, each time, Purdue celebrated by sending out a saber-rattling press release.

"These dismissals strengthen our resolve to defend these cases vigorously and to the hilt," the company's top lawyer, Howard Udell, said. "We have not settled one of these cases, not one. Personal-injury lawyers who bring them in the hopes of a quick payday will continue to be disappointed."

During a speech in 2002, Purdue's chief spokesman, Robin

Hogen, described to fellow public-relations executives how the company had weathered the storm. "I have to admit that our company looked like food for about the first year of this crisis," said Hogen, whose taste for bow ties gave him the appearance of an aging prep-school boy. "We were quite reactive; we were kind of stunned. We were saying, well, look at the science, look at the data, read the literature. And we were trying to argue with scientific arguments in what became a political war. And we had to switch over to using more political consultants in fact."

Then Hogen teased his audience with the news that Purdue would soon announce the addition of a political "rock star" to its roster of advisers. "I can't tell you today who it is, but we're going to be bringing on a very impressive individual who is a political star," he said. "That's all that I can tell you—because it's a political issue. And we'd like to think that there's a level playing field out there somewhere and that science and truth will win the day. That, unfortunately, is not the truth, and, in fact, you have to be politically Machiavellian often to win the day. So that's the direction we are heading in."

That "rock star" was Rudolph W. Giuliani, the former mayor of New York City. Prior to the attacks of September 11, Giuliani had indeed had a Machiavellian political reputation. The grit and determination he displayed guiding a battered city back onto its feet tempered this image somewhat and led even his staunchest critics to praise him. There was speculation in 2002 that Giuliani would seek higher office. But he decided instead to cash in on his newfound stature by opening Giuliani Partners, a consulting firm. Drawing on his years as a hard-nosed federal prosecutor, Giuliani set himself up as a corporate "Mr. Clean" for hire. His clients included WorldCom, a telecom giant mired in an accounting scandal; the National Thoroughbred Racing Association, enmeshed in a bid-rigging controversy; and Merrill

Lynch, a Wall Street firm accused of misleading investors. Now he would help steer Purdue through the OxyContin crisis. Giuliani Partners didn't disclose its fees, but the services of the former New York mayor didn't come cheap. On the lecture circuit, he commanded $100,000 for an after-dinner talk.

In 2002, Giuliani had recently recovered from prostate cancer, and he frequently used his experience as a patient when speaking publicly about Purdue.

"There are tens of millions of Americans suffering from persistent pain," Giuliani said. "We must find a way to ensure access to appropriate prescription pain medications for those suffering from the debilitating effects of pain while working to prevent the abuse and diversion of these same vital medicines."

Purdue soon took advantage of Giuliani's political connections as well. Not long after Giuliani was hired, he and Bernard Kerik, the ex–New York City police commissioner, who had followed his boss into the private sector, contacted the head of the DEA, Asa Hutchinson. Along with its probe into Laura Nagel's inquiry, the agency was also investigating thefts of OxyContin from a Purdue manufacturing plant in New Jersey, and Kerik had been assigned to beef up security procedures at the facility.

"The mayor and I just met with Asa Hutchinson, the director of the DEA, his staff, and people from Purdue," Kerik, who would later be imprisoned on tax-fraud charges, told a reporter. "We don't want Purdue put in a position where it winds up being taken over by the courts. Or they get put out of business. What I'd like to see come out of this is we set model security standards for the industry."

The growing number of contacts between Giuliani and Hutchinson, a former senator from Arkansas, created consternation within the DEA. It's very unusual for the DEA's administrator to get directly involved in an agency investigation of a drug manufacturer. The Justice Department takes recommendations from the DEA field official handling the case and decides how to proceed. But once Giuliani was in the mix, the pace of the DEA inquiry at the Purdue plant slowed, as Hutchinson summoned subordinates to explain their reasons for continuing it.

Hutchinson, however, did not interfere with Laura Nagel's investigation and, in the spring of 2002, a DEA pharmacologist handed her a report that appeared to contain the type of bombshell she wanted to drop on Purdue. The pharmacologist, David Gauvin, had spent months hunched inside his tiny office cubicle, sifting through the 1,300 separate death reports that medical examiners had sent to the DEA in response to the agency's request for data on fatal oxycodone-related overdoses. Gauvin discarded 350 reports as not substantial enough for his analysis. He then extracted data from the remaining 950, in order to determine how often OxyContin had been the source of the oxycodone found during the autopsies or toxicological examinations of overdose victims.

Nagel had suspected that the percentage would be high. But Gauvin's findings exceeded her expectations. His analysis showed that OxyContin was certain or very likely to have been involved in one-half of all overdose deaths in his sample. To arrive at that figure, he broke fatalities into groups. One of these was labeled "OxyContin verified," because medical reports or police information showed evidence of an OxyContin tablet or prescription in relationship to the body. Another category, "OxyContin likely," included toxicology tests that detected oxycodone but not aspirin or acetaminophen—the over-the-counter analgesics found in traditional painkillers but not in OxyContin. Some 145 cases, or about 15 percent of those he reviewed, were classified as "Oxy-Contin verified," while another 318 deaths, or 34 percent of the cases he analyzed, were "OxyContin likely."

The statistics were sobering. But Nagel was most struck by another of Gauvin's conclusions. It was one, she believed, that could change the entire debate over OxyContin. In addressing the drug's abuse, Purdue executives had insisted that the pain-killer did not pose any risks to patients if used as directed by a doctor. But Gauvin had concluded from his research that patients properly prescribed OxyContin were also dying from over-doses.

He based that finding on autopsy reports showing that over-dose victims often had a mix of prescription drugs in their systems when they died. Such results weren't unusual. It was rare for an overdose death to involve a single medication, and the presence of only one drug typically indicated that a person had committed suicide by taking a large number of one kind of pill. What caught Gauvin's attention was the particular combination of medications in autopsy reports. Many of the overdose accounts he examined showed that victims also had traces of tran-quilizers and antidepressants in their blood. Gauvin knew that doctors frequently prescribed those medications to pain patients taking oxycodone to help them cope with anxiety, and, to him, the finding indicated that patients taking OxyContin were over-dosing. Nagel thought the results were so significant that the agency issued a press release summarizing Gauvin's findings and their apparent implications for patients. It read:

A "normal" patient receiving a standard OxyContin prescription regimen approved by the Food and Drug Administration may be a poly-drug user. One treatment strategy recommended for "chronic pain" patients is

the co-administration of opioids with antidepressants—
again, a treatment strategy [that], by its design, results
in poly-drug usage. With these facts in mind it was not
surprising to find that many of the OxyContin deaths
were associated with poly-drug toxicologies. This does
not minimize the significance of OxyContin in these
deaths.

Nagel was confident that FDA officials, when confronted with
the DEA data, would be forced into greater action. But when
Purdue executives and FDA officials showed up at her office to
examine the study, Nagel's bombshell blew up in her face.

Purdue officials quickly dismissed Gauvin's conclusion, saying that there was nothing in the data to scientifically support
the suggestion that pain patients were overdosing. Instead, they
pointed out, drug abusers often took different medications together to customize a high, and the combination of OxyContin
and a tranquilizer such as Xanax was a particularly popular mix.
A top FDA official at the meeting, Dr. Cynthia McCormick,
agreed and added that the death reports reviewed by the DEA
were too ambiguous to merit any conclusions about the safety of
OxyContin. "We don't believe there is cause for panic," another
FDA official concluded.

Nagel had been caught out of her depth. As a cop, she had
viewed the death data simplistically, but the picture it offered
was murkier. Years later, some of Gauvin's findings would prove
accurate—a mix of opioids and tranquilizers could prove deadly
for pain patients and abusers alike—but in 2002 he had leapt to
a conclusion that his data couldn't support. "It was the worst day
of my life," Nagel would later say.

Soon another threat to Purdue's profits and OxyContin sales
was extinguished, this time thanks to politics and the ambitions

of a company critic, Florida's state attorney general, Bob Butterworth. In 2001, Butterworth, whose state was an epicenter of
OxyContin abuse, had announced the opening of an investigation into Purdue, which had two objectives. One of the inquiry's
goals, Butterworth declared, was to determine if Purdue had im-
properly promoted OxyContin. The other goal, he said, was to
determine if company executives had told the truth when they
claimed in Congress that they had only become aware of Oxy-
Contin's abuse in early 2000. Butterworth cited the large number
of OxyContin-related deaths in Florida as the impetus for his
investigation. "I got involved primarily because I was reading
the reports of the deaths from the medical examiners," he told a
newspaper, the *South Florida Sun Sentinel*. "That sort of gets
your attention."

Butterworth could be a formidable foe. A few years earlier, he
had been in the forefront of state attorneys general nationwide
who launched a legal assault against the tobacco industry. But in
this case, Butterworth's inquiry was short-lived and lackluster.
Attorneys in his office obtained the names of about one hundred
former and present Purdue sales reps who could serve as key
witnesses in the inquiry. But a state investigator working for
Butterworth's office formally interviewed only one of the reps, a
man named William Gergely, who once had been Purdue's district sales manager for Pennsylvania and West Virginia. In that
interview, Gergely, who had been fired by Purdue in 2000 after a
colleague filed a sexual-harassment claim against him, offered
up potentially explosive information. He said that two senior
Purdue marketing executives had described OxyContin during a
meeting with sales reps as "non-habit-forming" and explained
that the weekend-long pain-management seminars sponsored
by the drugmaker were really "junkets" that Purdue had used to
recruit doctors as paid speakers to boost OxyContin sales.

But that's where the investigation ended. Butterworth was blocked by term limits from seeking another term as Florida's attorney general, so he decided to run for a seat in the state's legislature. With that election looming, he faced pressure to close open investigations, both to gain the political benefit from a resolution and to eliminate any risk that the next attorney general would shut it down. In November 2002, just four days before Floridians went to the polls, Butterworth and Purdue announced they had struck a deal to end the state probe. Purdue agreed to pay $2 million to Florida to help the state underwrite the costs of a prescription-monitoring system. In exchange, Butterworth closed his investigation. A few days later, he was soundly defeated in the election.

Not long afterward, on New Year's Day 2003, Lindsay Myers lay in a hospital room in Johnson City, Tennessee, screaming in pain. A few hours later, she gave birth to a son. He was healthy and weighed six pounds and eleven ounces. His first name was Brennon, but Lindsay and Jane started calling him by his middle name, Kyle. Jane, realizing she would need to take care of Kyle, set up a crib, a changing table, and toys in her bedroom and brought him home to Pennington Gap from the hospital.

The months before Kyle's birth had been desperate ones for Lindsay and her parents. She was hooked on OxyContin again and was using a credit card from her father to cover the cost of filling up her friends' cars with gas. In return, they gave her cash, which she then spent on drugs.

Lindsay thought about having an abortion, and several times she made an appointment at a nearby abortion clinic but never showed up. Her drug use increased along with her fears about having a baby. Larry Lavender, the drug-abuse counselor, who had been working with Lindsay for months, worried that she might end up dead. Her parents were also in a panic, and Lavender suggested to Jane and Johnny that it might be best, given their daughter's fragile state, to put her into a long-term residential treatment program until her pregnancy was over. They agreed, and Lavender found a facility in Chattanooga, Tennessee, that took in pregnant women.

Jane and Johnny drove Lindsay to the clinic, where they were told that she would be kept on methadone until the baby was born. This was standard medical practice, as it prevented an expectant mother from undergoing the stresses of withdrawal prior to childbirth. But Jane got scared that Lindsay's baby would be born dependent on opioids and decided to bring her back to Pennington Gap.

By now Lindsay had a new boyfriend, with whom she was living. And one day, when Jane went to see her, he said that Lindsay was in jail—a few hours earlier, she had been arrested at a local Walmart for shoplifting vials of nasal spray. Lindsay was bailed out, but she kept stealing to support her habit. Expensive jewelry started to disappear from her family's home, including a diamond-studded ring that belonged to her father, her brother's gold rope necklace, and an emerald ring with diamonds that belonged to her mother.

Larry Lavender got a tip that Lindsay was pawning the jewelry at a local video store. He passed the information on to Jane, who went down to the store and started buying the pieces back. Her parents gave Lindsay a choice: After she gave birth, she could either go into a residential treatment program or they would have her prosecuted for stealing family jewelry.

A few weeks after Kyle was born, Lindsay left home for the Hazelden Clinic, the well-known substance-abuse treatment facility in Minnesota. After a successful month of treatment there, she moved to Phoenix, Arizona, where she lived in a halfway house. While on the phone with her mother, Lindsay wondered whether she should come back to Lee County or if she and Kyle should start a new life somewhere else.

Several months later, Lindsay came home to see Kyle and her parents. Her recovery appeared to be going well, but she told Jane that she had decided she couldn't take care of Kyle, at least for now. She had a job waiting for her back in Phoenix and was going to counseling meetings just about every night. She wanted to start college in the fall. Being a single mom on top of it all, she told her mother, would be too much.

Johnny agreed to drive her back to Arizona in her Jeep. Jane didn't think Lindsay would really go, but she and Johnny were prepared to legally adopt Kyle. While Lindsay packed, Jane kept waiting for her daughter to announce that she had changed her mind. When Lindsay was done, Johnny loaded her bags into the Jeep. Jane listened as the car started down the hill, away from the house. She expected to hear the car stop and back up. It didn't.

FOR MONTHS, Purdue executives had celebrated as critics and adversaries such as Laura Nagel and Art Van Zee fell by the way-side or got steamrolled by its public-relations machine. But in December 2002, Purdue executives received a notice that threw a damper on that mood. It was a subpoena from the office of the United States Attorney for the Western District of Virginia— the federal prosecutor's office in Roanoke, where Gregory Wood, the health-care investigator, worked—notifying Purdue that the Department of Justice had formally opened an investigation into the company's marketing of OxyContin.

During the previous months, two assistant U.S. Attorneys had come to share Gregory Wood's interest in the false marketing claims that Purdue sales reps had made for OxyContin, and they began to wonder if higher-ups in the company had orchestrated that campaign. The two men, Rick Mountcastle, a stocky ex-Marine, and the tall and somber-looking Randy Ramseyer, worked out of a satellite facility in Abingdon, Virginia, a small, quaint city in the foothills of the Appalachians located about 130 miles west of the U.S. Attorney's main office in Roanoke. Their offices were located in a small strip mall right around the corner from the neat brick building on Abingdon's main street that housed the federal court.

In the years since Purdue had started marketing OxyContin, Mountcastle and Ramseyer, like other law-enforcement officials, had seen the mix of cases they handled change drastically. By 2001, virtually all of them—robberies, fraud, assaults, and pill-mill cases—had a connection to Purdue's drug.

In late 2002, just before Bob Butterworth closed his investigation, an assistant state prosecutor in his office named Jody Collins had sent a letter to a Purdue lawyer, demanding documents about one of the key questions Butterworth had wanted answered: When had Purdue first learned about OxyContin's abuse and what had the company done? Because the Florida case settled, Collins never got answers to her questions. Mountcastle and Ramseyer intended to find them.

TEN

A Reckoning

THE MORNING OF MAY 10, 2007, BROKE BRIGHT AND BLUE over Abingdon, a onetime junction town trains passed through on their way to Appalachian coal mines. By 2007, its pleasant main street was dotted with restored Colonial-era houses and landmarks such as the Barter Theatre, a playhouse founded during the Great Depression, where local farmers could exchange produce for the price of an admission ticket. Not far from the Barter stood another historical landmark, a large, elegant mansion that once housed the venerable Martha Washington College for Women. It was now a hotel, the Martha Washington Inn, and on that May morning, three top executives of Purdue—Michael Friedman, Howard Udell, and Dr. Paul Goldenheim—emerged from the building to face a day of reckoning they had never believed would arrive.

Eight years had passed since OxyContin had made its mark in places like Lee County. Since then, the drug's use and abuse had spread throughout the United States, affecting and claiming thousands of lives. The ranks of its victims included not just rural Americans but also urban residents, the well heeled, and the well known. In 2003, conservative radio commentator Rush

Limbaugh, who liked to rail against drug abusers as weak and morally bankrupt, admitted that he too was addicted to Oxy-Contin.

Overdose deaths involving legal opioids had continued to rise at an alarming rate, growing in lockstep with the number of prescriptions written by doctors. The "war on pain" was still in full swing. In 2001, a group that set standards for hospitals, the Joint Commission on the Accreditation of Healthcare Organizations, adopted pain as the "fifth vital sign." The action, which followed lobbying by companies like Purdue and opioid advocates, encouraged healthcare providers to ask patients about their level of pain and to treat it, often with opioids. Hospital patients were also given survey forms and asked to rate doctors on the adequacy of their pain treatment, prompting doctors to prescribe more pills.

Some physicians, alarmed by the public controversy over OxyContin, had switched to alternative medications such as methadone, which, along with its use in addiction treatment, is prescribed to treat pain. But methadone can also be lethal, particularly in the hands of someone who is unaware of how it works. Methadone does not produce a high as quickly as oxycodone and lingers in the body for far longer, making it likely that an inexperienced user, waiting for a quick rush, will take more of it and overdose. As the demand for painkillers mounted, manufacturers of pills containing oxycodone or hydrocodone started sending huge quantities to hot spots where OxyContin abuse had been rampant. Mexican drug cartels, recognizing America's growing appetite for opioids, began to produce massive quantities of cheap heroin for shipment into the United States.

As the scope of the opioid epidemic took shape, federal officials and professional groups such as the American Medical Association did little, if anything, to stem the tide. Even sensible recommendations from pain-treatment specialists aimed at protecting patients and the public were ignored or opposed. One idea was to require doctors to undergo a few hours of mandatory training to be able to prescribe the potentially most addicting medications such as OxyContin. In 2001, the FDA had adopted a rule that required doctors to undergo brief training if they wanted to use a new addiction-treatment drug called buprenorphine. A pain expert, Dr. Nathaniel Paul Katz, thought it was absurd that doctors were required to receive training to prescribe a medication to treat addiction but only needed to fill out minor paperwork to receive a DEA license to prescribe drugs that could addict. Katz, who was an adviser to the FDA, pushed for years to get a rule requiring mandatory training to prescribe the most powerful narcotics. But FDA officials never championed the proposal, and the American Medical Association bitterly opposed it as inconvenient for doctors.

Amid the turmoil, Purdue and its executives maintained that they had done nothing wrong and that the company's actions had always served a single goal—the interests of pain patients. But that charade was about to end.

Since sending Purdue its first subpoena in December 2002, Rick Mountcastle and Randy Ramseyer, along with a team of federal prosecutors and investigators, had spent four years plowing through thousands of internal Purdue emails, records, and other documents. They called former Purdue sales reps, marketing executives, researchers, medical officers, and chemists to testify under oath before a federal grand jury, which met inside the courthouse in Abingdon. Doctors who prescribed OxyContin to their patients and pharmacists who filled those prescriptions described to grand jurors how they discovered that claims made to them by Purdue sales reps had turned out to be false. FDA officials also testified about what Purdue had told them and about what the company had never revealed.

A doctor from Indiana, Stephen L. Baker, described to grand jurors how a company sales rep had claimed to him that Oxy-Contin, because it was a long-acting medication, was safer than drugs like Percocet and that addicts would suffer strokes and heart attacks if they injected it. Another Indiana physician recalled how a Purdue sales rep had urged him to switch patients benefiting from other medications to OxyContin because it was "clearer and less addicting." He had also gotten a letter in June 2000 from that rep claiming that the medical use of powerful opioids like OxyContin posed a patient addiction risk of less than 1 percent, the same baseless figure that David Haddox liked to cite.

In a secret grand-jury session, Mark Ross, an ex–sales rep covering Tazewell County, Virginia, the site of one of the earliest outbreaks of OxyContin abuse, testified that he repeatedly warned his managers that the waiting room of a local doctor was filled with obvious drug seekers and abusers. His Purdue bosses, Ross explained, told him he was paid to sell drugs, not to determine if a doctor was running a pill mill.

Prosecutors also subpoenaed the Purdue sales officials who covered the pain clinic in Myrtle Beach, South Carolina, that the DEA shut down in mid-2001. Purdue had once attributed the boom in OxyContin prescriptions written there to the area's aging population. But company sales officials admitted in their testimony that they long suspected the clinic was a pill mill and were aware that state officials had suspended the medical license of its owner, Dr. David M. Woodward. Still, a Purdue district manager had recommended that Woodward, who directed how doctors he hired at his clinic prescribed drugs, undergo training as a paid speaker for Purdue. Another doctor, discovering he was scheduled to speak alongside Woodward at a Purdue-sponsored conference, refused to go on and described him, according to a sales official's testimony, as a "sociopath" who traded drugs for sex with patients. Two years after the DEA shut down his clinic, Woodward received a fifteen-year prison sentence.

The team headed by Ramseyer and Mountcastle worked on the OxyContin case with single-minded purpose—at one point, Ramseyer was diagnosed with cancer and took a break to undergo treatment, before returning to the investigation. The inquiry was so all-consuming that the Justice Department had to deputize Virginia state prosecutors to handle other cases in the Abingdon court, because federal lawyers were consumed by the OxyContin investigation. One of those deputized was Dennis Lee, the prosecutor from Tazewell County who had met in 2000 with Purdue executives to alert them to the devastation OxyContin was causing there. Unknown to Lee, that meeting took place right about the same time that Purdue sales managers were telling Mark Ross to ignore signs that doctors in Tazewell County were prescribing OxyContin to drug seekers and addicts.

In going through subpoenaed Purdue documents, federal prosecutors also uncovered how the company misrepresented data to overcome the biggest roadblock to OxyContin sales—physician concerns about the drug's addictive potential. Some of that information was contained in a chart used by sales reps eager to convince doctors that OxyContin was more stable in a patient's bloodstream than a traditional narcotic and so would not produce the same rush. The FDA had told Purdue that data was bogus, but the company trained its reps to use it anyway.

In other cases, prosecutors discovered, Purdue had concealed information from regulators. Some of that data related to another claim the drug agency allowed Purdue to make when it first started marketing OxyContin: that patients taking less than 60 milligrams daily of the drug—a relatively low dose—could stop it abruptly without going through the anxiety and discomfort associated with opioid withdrawal. Purdue sales reps used the claim as another tool to allay physician concerns that Oxy-Contin could produce serious dependence or addiction in a patient.

The FDA had allowed the claim based on the results of a Purdue-funded study that reported such patients exhibited "no overt withdrawal syndrome." But prosecutors discovered that by 2000 Purdue had begun receiving calls from patients on low doses, who were experiencing significant withdrawal symptoms. Soon, Purdue officials were sending one another emails about the "risk management" implications if the study's findings were inaccurate.

In 2001, a Purdue researcher, after investigating the study's underlying data, concluded that 25 percent of patients exhibited symptoms consistent with withdrawal. Purdue's medical department started telling doctors who called the company that patients needed to be slowly tapered off OxyContin to avoid withdrawal. But prosecutors found emails showing that the company allowed sales reps to give the questionable study to doctors, apparently with the blessing of senior executives. A 2003 email written by a top Purdue regulatory-affairs official indicated that Michael Friedman, Howard Udell, and Paul Goldenheim had approved the decision. "Howard, Michael, and Paul agree that the following two literature articles can be disseminated in a low key fashion by our sales force," that email stated. "There is to be no highlighting in these articles prior to leaving them behind, they are not to be disseminated [sic] at conventions and/or in booths but to be used in an appropriate manner with individual physicians."

Meanwhile, other internal Purdue emails showed that some medical officers thought the company needed to notify the FDA about the withdrawal issue, asking whether "we want to say: Dear regulatory authority: we no longer think it is correct to say that you can abruptly . . . stop therapy at 20–60 mg/day without risk" of withdrawal. One Purdue researcher wrote, "We think that tapering of dose is the more prudent medical recommendation," and added, "P.S. If we know one of our issued study reports is wrong, it should be a priority to correct it and file an amended report." In grand-jury testimony, FDA officials said the agency never got that report.

During their inquiry, prosecutors also came across emails indicating that senior executives of Purdue learned about wider abuse of OxyContin well before they said they did. And they heard about a former Purdue employee that worked under Howard Udell in the company's legal department who could offer an eyewitness account.

Prosecutors learned about the woman, Maureen Sara, from Paul Hanly, a plaintiffs' lawyer specializing in product-liability cases. By 2005, Hanly and his partner, who were based in New York, were handling a large numbers of cases against Purdue. Sara had herself become addicted to OxyContin following a back injury she sustained in a car accident and was among their clients.

When Hanly interviewed her, Sara recounted a story with potentially disastrous legal implications for Udell and other Purdue executives. She said that Udell asked her while she was working for him at Purdue in the late 1990s to go on the Internet and find chat rooms frequented by drug abusers, in order to see if they were discussing OxyContin. Those chat rooms were abuzz with people remarking how easy it was to crush OxyContin and abuse it. Sara said she told Udell what she was finding and that

he instructed her to continue her investigation and write a report. But when she delivered the report to him, Sara said, he
ordered her to get rid of it.

Sara was hardly an ideal witness. Along with her addiction to
OxyContin, she had gotten fired from Purdue, and she didn't
have any of the emails she said Udell and she had exchanged.
Nonetheless, Hanly contacted federal prosecutors in Virginia,
and Randy Ramseyer suggested that he accompany Sara to
Abingdon so she could testify before the grand jury. The trip
turned out to be a disaster. On the evening before her scheduled
testimony, Sara disappeared, and Hanly discovered her the following morning in the emergency room of an Abingdon hospital, where she'd gone to plead with doctors to give her painkillers.
Her grand-jury appearance was canceled, and Hanly returned to
New York convinced he had wasted his time. But in their memo,
prosecutors cited emails that backed up parts of Sara's story. In
June 1999, for instance, she sent Udell an email stating that her
Internet research had found "numerous discussions of misuse
and abuse of Purdue products, in particular OxyContin." A
month later, prosecutors said, she also forwarded to the Purdue
lawyer an email sent to the company by John Burke, a drug-
diversion investigator in Ohio. "I continue to see OxyContin increase in abuse with our doctor shoppers and sellers," Burke
wrote. "I suspected the trend was temporary, but it appears to be
a valid trend."

In their memo, prosecutors also cited testimony by Sara in
a deposition she gave during her lawsuit against Purdue. She
testified that she sent Udell an email in the fall of 1999, warning
that Purdue's plan to start selling a 160-milligram version of
OxyContin—a tablet twice as strong as the most powerful dose
then available—could have tragic consequences. "They are killing themselves with the 80s," she said her email stated. "Why

would we come out with a 160." Udell was irate, Sara testified, after getting her message, and said words to the effect of "What are you doing? If this comes out in discovery, we are screwed." He then ordered her to retrieve all copies of the email and destroy them, she said.

It wasn't unusual for the Justice Department to bring legal action against pharmaceutical companies. Starting in the late 1990s, federal prosecutors had begun to regularly sue drugmakers, typically charging a company with making a false advertising claim for a medication or for promoting it to doctors for use "off-label"—to treat a medical condition for which the FDA had not approved its use. (Doctors can prescribe a drug for any condition they think advisable, but companies can only promote it for FDA-approved purposes.)

But Mountcastle and Ramseyer decided early in their investigation that Purdue's violations far surpassed the typical case. They believed the company had acted criminally by training its sales representatives to misrepresent OxyContin's potential for abuse and addiction. They also concluded that three senior company executives—Udell, Friedman, and Goldenheim—were participants in the company's scheme and had misrepresented when they first learned of OxyContin's abuse. When their investigation ended in mid-2006, Mountcastle and Ramseyer recommended that the three men be indicted on serious charges that could send them to prison if convicted, including conspiracy to defraud the United States.

Their boss, John L. Brownlee, the U.S. Attorney for the Western District of Virginia, backed that hard-nosed approach. Brownlee, who had political ambitions, looked like a Hollywood casting agent's idea of a prosecutor. He came from a distinguished family. His father, "Les" Brownlee, was a Vietnam War veteran and a former Secretary of the Army. John Brownlee had also served in the military, and he appeared destined to follow a well-trodden path taken by Rudy Giuliani and other U.S. Attorneys into elective office.

Well before 2006, lawyers for Purdue had sought to convince senior Justice Department officials that an investigation into the company was unwarranted. In 2004, for example, Brownlee and his team of prosecutors were summoned to Washington to meet with James Comey, who was then the deputy Attorney General of the United States. But when Comey walked into the meeting room, he had a single question. "Why are you prosecuting the chicken guy?" he asked. After it was explained to him that the case was against Purdue Pharma, a drugmaker, not Frank Perdue, the chicken producer known from television ads, Comey encouraged Brownlee and his colleagues to continue their probe.

In the summer of 2006, prosecutors notified Purdue and the three executives about their findings and the charges they planned to seek. By then the company and its executives had assembled an all-star legal team. Its members included a former U.S. Attorney in Manhattan, Mary Jo White, who represented Howard Udell; an experienced ex–federal prosecutor, Howard Shapiro, who represented Purdue; and Rudy Giuliani, who served as the team's adviser.

Defense lawyers worked to convince prosecutors that their conclusions were wrong and that they had cherry-picked documents to create a case that would quickly fall apart if tested in court. Over the course of a two-day period in September 2006, for example, they put on an eight-hour presentation for Brownlee and his team to rebut their allegations. Defense lawyers offered statements from several law-enforcement officials and a top FDA regulator, who said that they had been unaware of any significant abuse of OxyContin prior to early 2000, the time when Purdue executives said they'd learned about the problem.

The defense team had also reviewed internal Purdue emails and they showed ones to prosecutors that, they argued, demonstrated that company executives were taken by surprise when the U.S. Attorney in Maine issued his alert. In addition, they insisted that Purdue had reacted responsibly to the crisis and done everything possible to curb the drug's abuse.

Prosecutors knew that the men would vehemently reject any suggestion that they had intended to mislead lawmakers or anyone else. They also anticipated that defense lawyers would claim at a trial that the executives' statements to Congress weren't intended to imply that they were unaware of any reports of the drug's misuse, because some abuse of a narcotic was inevitable. Instead, they would argue that reports received by Purdue had not risen to a "significant" or "unusual" level, terms the men had used.

But prosecutors believed they had plenty of evidence to show otherwise, and in late September 2006 they sent a 120-page memo to John Brownlee containing recommendations for indictments, which was then forwarded to officials at Justice Department headquarters for review and approval.

At the Justice Department, middle-level staffers supported the move to indict the executives. But the Purdue team found a more receptive audience among senior department officials, who then included Bush Administration political appointees. A series of discussions took place between aides to the head of the department's criminal division, Alice S. Fisher, and defense lawyers, in which John Brownlee and other officials who supported indictments did not participate. Rudy Giuliani, then seen as a potential Republican candidate in the upcoming presidential election, also took part in the talks.

On October 11, two weeks before prosecutors were scheduled to seek grand-jury indictments, a major meeting was held at the

Justice Department, at which defense lawyers, Alice Fisher, John Brownlee, and other department officials were present. Defense lawyers put on a presentation similar to the one they had given to Brownlee and his team. But by then a decision had apparently been made. Top department officials made it clear that they believed that felony charges against the Purdue executives were not justified.

Plea bargaining soon began. It was agreed that Purdue, as a company, would plead guilty to a felony charge known as "misbranding" and admit it had, among other things, deceptively promoted OxyContin as less likely to produce abuse and addiction than traditional painkillers. Under the agreement, the three executives would each plead guilty to a single misdemeanor charge of "misbranding." The misdemeanor violation, which was also cited in the prosecution memo, was an unusual one, because it allowed the Justice Department to hold Friedman, Udell, and Goldenheim liable, as Purdue's responsible corporate officers, for crimes committed by their subordinates, without prosecutors having to show that the men participated in those actions or knew about them. It was also agreed that the three men, who all insisted they had done nothing wrong, would be sentenced to perform community service rather than go to jail.

In late October 2006, just hours before the plea deal was to be signed, it almost fell apart. John Brownlee received a late-night phone call from a top aide to the Justice Department's deputy attorney general, Paul McNulty. During the call, that aide, Michael J. Elston, urged Brownlee to delay finalizing the plea agreement, because Howard Udell's lawyer, Mary Jo White, wanted more time to discuss it. Brownlee later testified that he told Elston he found his call inappropriate.

"I told him to go away and he did," Brownlee said.

Months later, on that clear May morning in 2007, Friedman,

Udell, and Goldenheim made the short walk from the Martha
Washington Inn to the federal courthouse in Abington. Inside
the courtroom, they each pled guilty to a single charge of "misbranding." Afterward, they were escorted into the building's
basement, where they were photographed and fingerprinted before being released. As a corporate jet flew them back to Connecticut, Brownlee held a press conference in Roanoke. He
announced that Purdue, as a company, had agreed to pay $600
million in fines and penalties to settle the charges against it and
highlighted the guilty pleas by the executives, who also agreed to
pay $34.5 million in fines. Their pleas also meant the three men
now had criminal records, a history that would bar them for
years from holding an executive position with any drug company that did business with the federal government. But within
minutes of Brownlee's announcement, defense lawyers went on
the offensive, arguing that the executives had done nothing
wrong and that the charge to which they had pled guilty had not
required the government to prove that they had.

Prosecutors did not suggest any wrongdoing by any of the
Sacklers. But during the years in which the investigation unfolded, several family members who worked at Purdue stepped
back from their operational roles. In 2003, Richard Sackler resigned his post as president and became co-chairman of the
company's board. In May 2007, Dr. Kathe Sackler and Jonathan
Sackler ended their service as senior vice presidents and Mortimer D. A. Sackler relinquished his post as a vice president.
They all remained company directors.

In July 2007, the federal courthouse in Abingdon was packed
with parents who had lost children to OxyContin-related overdoses. They had come from as far away as Florida and California
to see whether or not the court would accept the plea agreement.
But the hearing's outcome was preordained: Its presiding judge,

James P. Jones, absent startling new information, was bound to approve it.

Hoping the judge would be swayed by their stories and send the three men to prison, parent after parent rose to tell of unimaginable grief that followed the discovery that a son or daughter had died of an OxyContin overdose. Some addressed the executives directly.

"You are responsible for a modern-day plague," one parent told them. "It is killing our children every day."

"I feel that you are illegal drug dealers," said another, "nothing more than a large corporate drug cartel. You created this drug, you promoted it, you pushed it, you lied about it, you even had the ex-mayor of New York City defend it. You have killed and continue to kill our future of tomorrow. You killed my son and so many others and continue to do so as I speak."

Then a woman rose and held up a small vial. She told the court that it contained the cremated ashes of her son. "Reject the plea agreement," the woman beseeched Judge Jones. "Money means nothing to them. Let the punishment fit the crime."

Randy Ramseyer told Judge Jones that the Justice Department believed the plea agreement was fair because it would send a message to other pharmaceutical-industry executives that they would be held to account. "To my knowledge, never before have pharmaceutical corporate officers been held criminally liable for this type of conduct," Ramseyer said. "It's unprecedented and it will reaffirm to executives in the pharmaceutical industry that they are held to higher standards because the products they deal with have such a high potential for endangering public safety."

But Ramseyer, apparently angered that efforts to indict the company's executives had failed, could not resist taking a shot at them.

"Wouldn't it be nice if the company's attorney would come to the podium and say Purdue is sorry for the crime it committed and sat down?" he said. "Wouldn't it be nice if the individuals' attorneys would come to the podium and say they're sorry they've breached that high standard that they've been entrusted to protect public safety, and then sit down. Everyone here knows that's not going to happen. When I sit down, the next public-relations campaign will begin for Purdue. They will attempt to minimize the crimes to which they have pled guilty. They will argue that they have done much good. They will argue that they are the only ones who care about pain management. They'll talk about their quote, unquote 'extraordinary efforts to stop abuse and diversion,' not because it has anything to do with this case; it's all done for public-relations reasons."

When Ramseyer sat down, defense lawyers painted the company's crimes as the result of a few renegade sales reps within it and portrayed Friedman, Udell, and Goldenheim as unwitting victims. "Committing or condoning misconduct, or causing harm, or letting harm occur to any person, is the antithesis of what Mr. Udell and his life are about," said Mary Jo White. "He is a high-minded and thoroughly ethical person who holds himself to the highest standards of conduct." A lawyer for Paul Goldenheim, who'd left Purdue in 2004, struck a similar note. "Dr. Goldenheim is in agony," his attorney, Andrew Good, said. "He has been in agony since this whole case began, because he is anything but a person who would tolerate that any harm should come to any person from what he has done."

When the long hearing drew to a close, Judge Jones spoke. In a booming voice, he told the court that he was troubled by his inability to send the executives to prison. But he added that his hands were tied by the terms of the plea deal. He placed the three executives on three years of probation and ordered them to perform four hundred hours of service in a drug-abuse or drug-treatment program.

The sun was still shining when those attending the hearing emerged from the courthouse. A small group of them held an impromptu rally, lifting up posters with pictures of lost children. Art Van Zee wanted to attend the hearing but was too busy with patients. But Sister Beth Davies had made the seventy-five-mile drive over from Pennington Gap. As she stood outside the court-room, she felt a mixture of satisfaction and regret.

"We didn't get want we wanted," Sister Beth said. "But at least they didn't get away with everything."

A few weeks later, John Brownlee appeared before a congressional committee in Washington, D.C., where a veteran U.S. senator from Pennsylvania, Arlen Specter, questioned him about the Purdue settlement. Specter, who was a former district attorney in Philadelphia, was perplexed by what he viewed as the contradictory charges in the case. If Purdue, as a company, had committed a felony, why hadn't its executives gone to jail?

"The corporation does not act by itself. It is inanimate. It acts through people," Specter told Brownlee. "So are you saying that you couldn't identify the people?"

"I think it is fair to say that when we looked at the proof as to the corporate entity and we looked at the proof as to particular individuals, that proof tested out differently," Brownlee replied. "As you well know, a corporation can be held criminally liable for the actions of its agents."

Specter, who had voiced criticism of the settlement, cut off Brownlee and kept pressing him. "There is a total disconnect," he said. "Either you have a basis for saying that there is an intent to mislead or you do not. And if you have a basis for saying there is an intent to mislead, it is because individuals acted in a way which led you to that conclusion. And that being so, I do not see how you can have a conclusion that the individuals were not wrongdoers who deserved jail."

Brownlee and Specter went around on this issue for several minutes before Brownlee said, "The evidence in this case was reviewed by career prosecutors and investigators, and it was their judgment—and I agree with them—that under the evidence in this case, that the charging decisions, the felony for the company and the strict liability misdemeanors for the executives, were the appropriate charging decisions."

During their exchange, Specter also asked Brownlee whether the information gathered during the Purdue investigation could have supported more serious charges against its officials. In his response, the prosecutor said he could only speak to information made public as a result of the case's resolution, because federal law barred him from disclosing other evidence gathered during the government's investigation.

Much of that evidence was contained in the 120-page memo prosecutors sent to Brownlee in September 2006. It also provided a detailed road map of what federal investigators discovered during their four-year journey inside Purdue. When the case was settled, the memo and the evidence within it were sealed and forgotten. Years later they would finally emerge, replete with dozens of emails exchanged between Purdue officials as the OxyContin crisis unfolded, including ones sent by company executives to members of the Sackler family.

It is impossible to know exactly what would have happened if the Justice Department had put the company and its executives on trial. But one thing is clear: It wouldn't have made a difference who won the case or who lost it.

What would have mattered is that the evidence, painstakingly gathered by prosecutors, would have been put on public display.

As the case played out in the Abingdon courthouse, witnesses would have testified and internal Purdue documents would have been entered as evidence. Whatever rebuttals defense lawyers offered, a bright light, both shocking and clarifying, would have shone on the actions of Purdue. That light would have illuminated the origins of the opioid epidemic and likely altered its course, sparing thousands of lives that would soon be lost.

ELEVEN

Empire of Deceit

IN 2018, AN OPIOID EPIDEMIC THAT BEGAN TWO DECADES earlier with OxyContin finally seized the nation's attention. Over 250,000 Americans had died from overdoses involving prescription painkillers. Every day, hospital emergency rooms nationwide treated 1,000 people for abusing or misusing these drugs. Prescriptions written for narcotic painkillers—and overdoses associated with the drugs—had started to slowly decline. But counterfeit versions of fentanyl were rapidly driving up the overall numbers of overdose deaths.

President Donald J. Trump, pointing to the death toll, officially declared the opioid crisis a national emergency. In early 2018, he announced a plan that included increasing addiction treatment and reducing the medical use of opioids. In that same speech, Trump called for a tougher approach to drug dealers, including using the death penalty. It wasn't clear how his administration planned to fund its proposals to deal with the opioid crisis, but experts acknowledged that government officials had failed to stem an epidemic when they had had the chance. "We didn't get ahead of it; nobody got ahead of it," said Dr. Scott Gottlieb, appointed by President Trump to head the FDA.

Journalists also sought to give the opioid crisis a face, that of the Sackler family. In 2017, both *Esquire* magazine and *The New Yorker* magazine published lengthy accounts that depicted Raymond and Mortimer Sackler as corporate titans who made billions from OxyContin's marketing and opened the door to the public-health catastrophe that followed. The articles' timing led *The New York Times* to undertake a survey of twenty-one museums and institutions worldwide that had received funds from the Sacklers or family-run foundations, to learn if any of them would return the money given its connection to the notorious painkiller. None of them planned to do so.

It was also in 2017 that Raymond Sackler, the last remaining Sackler brother, died, at the age of ninety-seven. Faced with a new burst of attention, Raymond and Mortimer's adult children who had once worked at Purdue stood behind the family's traditional wall of silence. However, Arthur Sackler's daughter, Elizabeth, an art historian and trustee of the Brooklyn Museum in New York, was eager to put space between the money she had inherited from her father's promotion of drugs, such as Valium, and the fortunes that her uncles and their families had reaped from OxyContin. In a statement issued to a reporter writing about museums and Sackler money, she pointed out that her uncles had purchased her father's share of Purdue Frederick following his death in 1987, a decade before OxyContin was launched. By 2017, sales of OxyContin had exceeded $31 billion, but her wing of the Sackler family had never made a dime from the drug. "The opioid epidemic is a national crisis and Purdue Pharma's role in it is morally abhorrent to me," she said.

Though the federal prosecutor Randy Ramseyer predicted that the Purdue executives' guilty pleas would affect the behavior of other companies' officials, that was not the case. Between 2007 and 2012, the three biggest wholesalers of prescription drugs in the United States—McKesson, Cardinal, and AmerisourceBergen—shipped 780,000,000 pain pills containing oxycodone or hydrocodone to West Virginia, a state already rife with opioid addiction, a newspaper there reported. The volume represented a quantity large enough to supply every man, woman, and child in the state of West Virginia with 433 pills. Over that same five-year period, more than 1,700 people in West Virginia died from fatal overdoses involving prescription opioids. Meanwhile, as the opioid epidemic intensified, drug-industry lobbyists succeeded in 2016 in getting a law passed that made it harder for the DEA to block shipments of pain pills going to doctors or pharmacies suspected as illegal outlets for opioids, according to a report in *The Washington Post*.

It is often said that prosecutors fall in love with their cases. And it is not usual for supervisors to modify or reject their recommendations. But the Justice Department, in choosing not to charge Purdue's executives with felonies, left unanswered the most critical question in the government's case: When did Purdue first learn about OxyContin's abuse and what did company officials do about it?

Michael Friedman, Howard Udell, and Paul Goldenheim would insist before and after their guilty pleas that they learned of the problem in early 2000. And years afterward, a Purdue spokesman, when asked about the prosecutors' recommendations for indictments, pointed to John Brownlee's 2007 Senate testimony in which he described the strict liability charges against the men as "appropriate."

But government prosecutors and investigators involved in the Purdue inquiry saw it very differently. They believed they had uncovered Purdue's original sin, one so shocking and heartsickening that it trumped all the lies the company admitted telling. The OxyContin disaster should have never happened, prosecu-

tors believed, because Purdue knew by 1997—three years before
the Maine alert—that its "wonder" drug was being abused but
said nothing to warn doctors, patients, and the public. "Even as
the conspirators marketed OxyContin as less addictive, less
abusable and less divertable than other opioids, as early as 1997
they began receiving reports from health care providers and the
news media indicative of widespread abuse and diversion of
OxyContin," prosecutors wrote in their 2006 memo.

If prosecutors were right, it wouldn't have taken much for
Purdue to have sounded an early alarm. Company officials could
have shared what they were learning with regulators and lawmakers and decided together what actions were needed. Years
later, Purdue would have been applauded for preventing a catastrophe rather than castigated for causing one. Years later, no one
would have questioned the source of the Sacklers' wealth or
whether prestigious museums should be taking the family's
money.

But being forthright also carried a price. If regulators at the
FDA or lawmakers had learned early on about the drug's abuse,
then Purdue risked losing its unique labeling claim—the one celebrated by company officials as its "principal selling tool"—just
as the massive marketing campaign for OxyContin was starting.
Absent that claim, doctors would have viewed OxyContin with
the same caution as any another narcotic. It would not have produced billions in profits. It could never have served as the vehicle
to let Purdue, in Raymond Sackler's words, reach the moon.

All the evidence prosecutors had unearthed to make their case
was contained in the 2006 memo they sent to John Brownlee.
And much of that evidence was reburied when top Justice Department officials rejected their recommendation for indictments. In their memo, prosecutors detailed everything they

believed officials of Purdue had learned about the early abuse of OxyContin and its predecessor, MS Contin, and how company officials had allegedly painted a false picture while making statements in Congress and elsewhere. The memo stated:

> Had the conspirators provided Congress and their sales representatives with the truth, that is that PURDUE had been aware, at least as early as 1997–1998, that both MS Contin and OxyContin were subject to widespread abuse and diversion but continued to market OxyContin as less addictive, abusable and subject to diversion in the face of this knowledge, the sales representatives would have lost all credibility with health care providers, and PURDUE's conduct would likely have been subject to much greater regulatory and Congressional scrutiny.

The memo cited dozens of internal Purdue emails, records, and other documents in support of those claims, starting with the extent of the company's knowledge of MS Contin's misuse. It had been far greater than the few "scattered" incidents that Purdue officials had claimed, prosecutors believed. And the company knew by 1996, internal Purdue emails showed, that addicts had discovered how to defeat MS Contin's time-release formulation in order to extract morphine from a tablet so they could shoot it up.

For example, in May of 1996, prosecutors found, Richard Sackler and Howard Udell were sent a medical-journal article about MS Contin abuse, called "Recovery of Morphine from a Controlled Release Preparation." And in August of that year, company records showed, a Purdue scientist assigned to research MS Contin abuse emailed his findings to Sackler, Udell, Michael Friedman, Paul Goldenheim, and other Sackler family members, including Raymond and Mortimer.

"I found MS Contin mentioned a couple of times on the internet underground drug culture scene," that researcher wrote in his email. "Most of it was mentioned in the context of MS Contin as a morphine source." He added he had also found an academic publication that mentioned "MS Contin as a source of morphine abuse in Australia."

The following year, Paul Goldenheim received a copy of an article from an American medical publication that reported, "Morphine is readily extracted from MS Contin for street abuse." And in another 1997 email, a top Purdue medical officer, Robert Kaiko, told company executives that MS Contin was the "most common source" of morphine for drug addicts in New Zealand. That year, Purdue executives were deciding whether to ask German drug regulators to place less-restrictive controls on sales of OxyContin sales there, but Kaiko pointed out in his email that the company would find that argument hard to make because it didn't have data about product abuse. "We do not have a post-marketing abuse monitoring system and database from which we could conclude that diversion/abuse is not occurring," he wrote.

By 1998, Purdue would get a better sense of that problem, when the *Canadian Medical Association Journal* published its study and an accompanying editorial warning that drug abusers would also seek out the company's latest time-release drug, Oxy-Contin. In March of that year, Howard Udell wrote a legal memo entitled "MS Contin Abuse," which he sent to members of the Sackler family involved in Purdue's operations. In the memo, the Purdue lawyer described several articles in Canadian newspapers that had appeared at around the same time as the study in the *Canadian Medical Association Journal*. He highlighted a passage from one of them, the *Ottawa Citizen,* which stated that "a prescription of 30 pain-killing morphine MS Contin 60-mg tablets—known as 'purple peelers'—cost $58 from a pharmacy but fetches [sic] $1,050 on the black market at $35 a tablet." He also noted in his memo that a virtually identical story had appeared on the front page of another Canadian newspaper, the *Vancouver Sun.*

By then Purdue officials also knew that OxyContin was being abused, an email found by federal investigators indicated. The email was written in the fall of 1997 by a senior Purdue marketing official, Mark Alfonso, and sent to Michael Friedman and other executives. In the memo, Alfonso reported that mentions of OxyContin were appearing on websites and in chat rooms frequented by drug abusers.

Monitoring that traffic, he wrote, "was enough to keep a person busy all day. We have three people that visit the site chat rooms. In addition, we have started a project that will have one of our people visit the most popular chat rooms at least once a month."

It was around that time, prosecutors believed, that Purdue officials, based on what they were learning about the abuse of OxyContin and MS Contin, should have called a time-out. But Purdue didn't do so, and it apparently showed no interest in telling doctors or even its own sales reps what it was learning about the vulnerability of its time-release drugs. Purdue apparently not only never alerted FDA officials about the *Canadian Medical Association Journal* study and its implications, but company sales reps kept giving out copies of the 1993 report by Dr. Daniel Brookoff, which suggested that drug abusers had little interest in time-release medications like OxyContin.

During 1999, the year before the Maine warning, prosecutors

found, Purdue received a flood of information about OxyContin abuse. That January, Howard Udell alerted a fellow company executive in an email that "We have in fact picked up references to abuse of our opioid products on the Internet." And that month a Purdue sales rep in Ohio reported in a call note that all one doctor there wanted to talk about was the "new street value of OxyContin."

By mid-1999, the tempo of reports coming into Purdue head-quarters intensified, prosecutors found. During a two-week period in August 1999, for example, Purdue executives were sent reports that a doctor in Pennsylvania had stopped writing pre-scriptions for OxyContin because his patients were altering them; that a Connecticut man had been arrested for trying to il-legally purchase OxyContin; that a Massachusetts man had told police that he preferred to crush the drug because it worked bet-ter "if he sniffs it"; and that a drugstore in Maryland had been robbed of OxyContin by armed thieves. Purdue's top officials also learned then that a Florida nurse was about to publish an article identifying OxyContin as a "drug of abuse," emails cited by federal investigators showed.

That same month, William Gergely, the only Purdue insider interviewed during the brief inquiry by Florida state attorney general Bob Butterworth, told his superiors that one doctor in his territory who was a "huge writer of OxyContin" had stopped prescribing all opioids after learning that some of his patients had been arrested for altering OxyContin prescriptions. And it was also at about this time that Purdue sales rep Kimberly Keith submitted her call notes about OxyContin's abuse in Lee County, Virginia, and that company officials became aware of the Oxy-Contin alert issued by Cambria County in the western part of Pennsylvania.

In September, soon after Maureen Sara sent Howard Udell

her email citing Internet chat-room discussions about Oxy-
Contin abuse, Friedman, Udell, and Goldenheim received two
similar emails from a Purdue employee, reporting chat-room
discussions about snorting OxyContin, according to records
found by investigators.

Still, Purdue did nothing, and many sales reps apparently
never learned about the extent of the drug's abuse. In their report, prosecutors cited a November 1999 memo sent by a Purdue district manager to reps in southwestern Virginia and West
Virginia—areas where abuse of OxyContin was exploding—
offering them tips about how to respond to concerns raised by
doctors. In it, he advised:

> Refer to studies involving over 20,000 patients that
> show less than 1% iatrogenic addiction when patients
> treated with opioids for pain. Doctor says, "they are
> crushing it and shooting it up"—say "how many of your
> patients come in with tracks on their arms?" Doctor
> responds none, then what's the issue? If he has some,
> should refer to addictionologist. Doctor says police
> arresting people sniffing crushed OxyContin—"Great!
> The police are doing their job. If the patients/abusers
> are reformulating it once they out your door, it's not
> your responsibility.

Just as that memo was going out, another newspaper, *The
Florida Times-Union*, published an article about the arrest of
a doctor in Jacksonville, Florida, on charges of running a pill
mill that sold OxyContin and other drugs. In it, a local law-
enforcement officer described the physician as "dealing prescription drugs to people just like a crack cocaine dealer would
be selling crack to people on the street."

An email written by the Purdue sales rep in Jacksonville quickly found its way to top company officials, prosecutors reported. "While many sales people have sold controlled release opioids as having less abuse potential, the current situation has placed us in an awkward situation," the rep wrote. "I feel we have a credibility problem with our product."

David Haddox, who had joined Purdue a few months earlier, also received the article from the Jacksonville paper. He apparently became concerned and he emailed company officials to suggest that Purdue implement a crisis-response plan, prosecutors found.

Michael Friedman replied that he didn't think such action was needed. "I simply do not want us to over-react to this specific story," he wrote in an email. "Physicians have been accused and arrested, from time to time, as long as these drugs have been around. This is not a repetitive pattern or something new. The case of one bad apple passes with time. I am concerned with long term issues that influence the use of these drugs, not one doctor who is dishonest."

Prosecutors saw more than a few "bad apples." Over the course of 1999, other physicians, including Dr. James Graves, the physician from Pace, Florida, had been arrested on charges of illegally dispensing OxyContin. Federal investigators also ran a search of call notes written by Purdue sales reps between 1997 and 1999 for the words "street value," "crush," and "snort," and reported that one or more of the terms appeared in 117 call reports written by reps in twenty-seven states.

Prosecutors also believed that executives at Purdue were concerned that the company's knowledge about how widely its painkillers were being abused might leak out. In June of 2000, a few months after the Maine alert, Mark Alfonso sent Michael Friedman an email describing how the chaos involving OxyContin reminded him of what he had observed earlier when he managed sales of MS Contin in the Midwest.

"I recall that I received this kind of news on MS Contin all the time, and from everywhere," Alfonso wrote. "Some pharmacies would not even stock MS Contin for fear they would be robbed. In Wisconsin, Minnesota and Oklahoma, we had physicians indicted for prescribing too much MS Contin." Friedman, prosecutors stated, forwarded Alfonso's email to Howard Udell with a message asking if the lawyer wanted "all this chat on e-mail?" A year later, Friedman, Udell, and Goldenheim all testified that they were aware of only a few scattered incidents of MS Contin abuse during the seventeen years the company marketed that drug.

Purdue was also worried about the potential damage posed by call notes written by sales reps, prosecutors asserted. So by 2001, company lawyers started training reps to avoid using words such as "addiction" and "abuse" in their notes.

The scope of the profits that Purdue executives and the Sacklers derived from OxyContin was extraordinary, prosecutors discovered. By 2002, six years after the drug appeared, its annual sales had reached $1.5 billion, or three times the revenue that MS Contin sales had produced during a decade. Within Purdue, the awarding of "salaries, bonuses, director's fees, and other similar payments" corresponded to the increase in OxyContin sales, prosecutors reported. They also found that in 2001 alone, companies controlled by Raymond Sackler and Mortimer Sackler or their families received $1 billion in profits. Those funds flowed into a thicket of Sackler-owned business entities with names such as BR Holdings Associates, Beacon Company, and Rosebay Medical Company, which were reminiscent of the paper corporate empires created by Arthur Sackler. Years later, in 2015, *Forbes* magazine welcomed the families of Raymond and

Mortimer Sackler as the latest newcomers to its list of the wealthiest Americans, with a fortune estimated at $14 billion. According to the magazine, they had edged out "storied families" such as the Mellons and Rockefellers in the magazine's rankings.

"How did the Sacklers build the 16th largest fortune in the country?" *Forbes* asked. "The short answer: making the most popular and controversial opioid of the 21st century—OxyContin."

The Sacklers might have fallen short of reaching that storied stature, however, if the Justice Department had gone to trial. Had the prosecutors' evidence been aired, doctors would likely have become more wary of claims by Purdue and other opioid makers and reduced their wholesale dispensing of the drugs. Had the government insisted on a trial, lawmakers and regulators might have turned a deaf ear to arguments by drug-industry lobbyists and their medical allies that succeeded in blocking reasonable controls on opioid use. Professional medical organizations, law-enforcement associations, and groups representing pain patients might have learned that drug companies such as Purdue don't give their money away without expectations and broken their dependency on industry funds.

If they needed evidence of such motives, these groups would have benefited from reviewing the transcript of a March 2001 telephone-answering-machine message contained in the prosecutors' memo. At the time, a newspaper had just published an article about a Medicaid investigation involving OxyContin, in which Connecticut state attorney general Richard Blumenthal expressed concerns about what he viewed as Purdue's overly aggressive marketing of the drug to doctors. The next morning, Purdue's chief spokesman, Robin Hogen, left a message on the phone of one of Blumenthal's assistants that made it clear that

Purdue used money to reward friends and withheld it to punish enemies.

"I wanted to signal our very high level of disappointment in the way the whole press was handled around the A.G.'s comments on this Medicaid fraud," Hogen said. "I thought we had an understanding he was going to clarify and retract the statements last night. The door was wide open, and he did not do it. Purdue Pharma is a significant supporter of the Democratic party. It's very unfortunate that this had to happen to one of your major benefactors. I think there's an election coming up, and I can assure you this has not helped his cause in this camp."

A few days later, a lawyer in Blumenthal's office sent copies of the tape and a certified transcript of Hogen's message to Raymond Sackler, Howard Udell, Michael Friedman, and Hogen. Both Udell and Hogen sent subsequent letters of apology.

As the opioid epidemic expanded, it was not only the Justice Department that failed to take desperately needed steps. Drug regulators, lawmakers, medical associations, and even public-health officials seemed frozen, uncertain of what to do or how to respond. They also seemed unable or unwilling to stand up against the drug industry even when those actions would have benefited patients. During the Obama Administration, for example, White House officials proposed a rule, suggested more than a decade earlier by Dr. Nathaniel Paul Katz, that would have required mandatory training for doctors prescribing powerful opioids like OxyContin. But lobbyists for the American Medical Association made it clear to administration officials that they would go to war over such a proposal, and the White House backed down.

Drugmakers paid little heed to the few rules that the FDA adopted to control the marketing of high-powered opioids. One small company, Insys Therapeutics, even borrowed pages from

Purdue's playbook to drive sales of its product, a form of fentanyl called Subsys. While the FDA approved the drug's use only for cancer sufferers, Insys sales data soon showed that such patients represented only 1 percent of the Subsys prescriptions written by doctors. The drug's biggest prescribers, it turned out, were not cancer experts but regular physicians, including several who would be charged with running pill mills. As with early heavy prescribers of OxyContin, some of those doctors also received tens of thousands of dollars in speaking fees from Insys. To spur sales, Insys adopted Purdue's bonus system in which reps were rewarded based on the increase in the dollar value of prescriptions their doctors wrote rather than an increase in the number of prescriptions. This created a system that paid the biggest bonuses to reps who promoted the strongest doses of Subsys.

In 2010, Purdue began to sell a new form of OxyContin, which the company said was more resistant to abuse. Art Van Zee had urged the company to take that step a decade earlier, but Purdue officials said it had taken them years to develop the required technology. It may have been a coincidence, but Purdue launched the product just as its patent on the original form of the painkiller was expiring. The company took a number of other steps to help curtail the opioid crisis, such as funding prescription-monitoring programs and helping to distribute naloxone, the drug used to reverse overdoses. Also, Purdue said that in 2016 it ended its long use of paid speakers to promote OxyContin.

But Purdue found it increasingly difficult to distance itself from the havoc sowed by OxyContin. In 2017, the United States Attorney's office in Connecticut began a new investigation into the company in response to a 2016 article in the *Los Angeles Times*. The *Times* reported that the company's claim that Oxy-Contin's analgesic effect lasted twelve hours was misleading and that in many patients it wore off more quickly. If so, patients would have had to take more OxyContin to get relief and this would place themselves at greater risk for dependency or addiction. In response to the article, Purdue insisted that OxyContin worked as claimed.

Dozens of states, cities, towns, and tribes of Native Americans had also filed a wave of new lawsuits against Purdue and other opioid manufacturers. In each case, the drug companies were under attack for reckless and misleading promotion of drugs that caused taxpayers to spend untold billions on healthcare costs related to drug abuse and addiction. Even the small Philadelphia suburb of Bensalem, where Michael Friedman first publicly testified to the extent of Purdue's knowledge of OxyContin's abuse, had sued the company.

In early 2018, with sales of OxyContin declining and without new major drugs in development, Purdue announced a major retrenchment. It would no longer send out sales reps to doctors' offices to promote OxyContin and was cutting back its sales staff to two hundred people—its approximate size before OxyContin was launched. Purdue was still promoting the drug overseas, but the company's decision was an acknowledgment that its glory days were behind it.

Some of those who had crossed swords with Purdue, like Terry Woodworth, the onetime DEA official, thought that moment should have come a decade earlier, when the federal government had Purdue on the ropes. But Justice Department officials balked when they had the opportunity and allowed the last, best chance to slow the opioid epidemic to slip away.

The War Against Pain Revisited

MUCH HAS HAPPENED SINCE THE FIRST PUBLICATION OF THIS book in 2003. But perhaps the biggest change involves a new understanding of the benefits and risks posed by powerful opioids such as OxyContin.

During the 1990s and 2000s, doctors were principally concerned about the threat such drugs posed for abuse and addiction. But over the past decade, a wealth of research has emerged to show that the long-term use of opioids, even when taken as directed, carries an array of patient risks such as emotional dependency, reduced sexual drive, extreme lethargy, increased falls in the elderly, and even the development of an increased sensitivity to pain. Just as important, a number of recent medical studies have shown that pain patients often recover faster, with fewer complications, if provided with treatments other than opioids.

As a result, the treatment of pain is again undergoing a sea change. Hospital emergency rooms no longer routinely use opioids, and patients recovering from surgery are given over-the-counter pain relievers rather than powerful narcotics. Doctors have also turned away from using opioids for specific conditions such as migraine headaches, and federal agencies are urging that opioids be employed only as a treatment of last resort.

This turnabout began quietly in 2003 with a little-noticed study in *The New England Journal of Medicine*. The report was written by Dr. Jane Ballantyne, who was then the head of pain treatment at one of this country's most prestigious hospitals, Massachusetts General in Boston. For years, Ballantyne had been a loyal soldier in the "war on pain," but she began to notice phenomena that troubled her. While chronic-pain patients put on opioids did well initially, their health, as measured in outcomes such as pain relief or improved physical function, soon flattened out or even regressed.

Their response reminded Ballantyne of what she had observed in hospital patients on mechanical ventilators who were sedated with opioids. Over time, as patients required higher opioid doses, they became more, not less, sensitive to pain. Some patients writhed in agony at the touch of a bedsheet against their skin.

Ballantyne believed such reactions were attributable to "tolerance," the natural phenomenon associated with opioids in which the body adapts to a drug and requires higher doses to maintain the same level of pain relief. During the height of the "war on pain," opioid advocates had insisted that tolerance was not a barrier to treating chronic pain, because doctors could increase dosages as high as needed, without ill effects, to overcome tolerance. But in her 2003 article, Ballantyne challenged this idea. By ramping up opioid doses, she warned, doctors ended up chasing pain and, in the process, risked harming patients. While "it was previously thought that unlimited dosage escalation was at least safe, evidence now suggests that prolonged, high-dose opioid therapy may be neither safe nor effective," she wrote.

Opioid proponents marked Ballantyne as a traitor. But subsequent research would support her warning as prescient. Researchers in Denmark—a country that keeps detailed records on how patients respond to differing medical treatments—found that pain patients put on non-drug treatments recovered at a rate four times faster than patients given opioids. Researchers with the U.S. Department of Veterans Affairs would report similar findings.

The damage inflicted on patients by the unbridled use of opioids became apparent in other ways. Studies have found that workers who were given high dosages of opioids to treat common injuries such as back pain were out of work three times longer than those who were put on a lower dosage, and some of them never returned to their jobs. Even insurers who had helped stoke the opioid boom by refusing to pay for other kinds of pain treatment began to have second thoughts, though these were likely attributable to financial concerns rather than worries about patient welfare. It turns out that the opioid-driven approach to pain was costing them far more than they imagined, in terms of both patient care and addiction treatment.

In recent years, pain specialists who championed high-dose opioid use have offered explanations for the failings of the "war on pain" or have tried to rewrite their roles in it. But their enthusiastic advocacy has produced a terrible legacy—a generation of "narcotized" patients who find it nearly impossible to give up their dependency on opioids and seek other methods of treatment.

"Addiction is not the real problem," one of those advocates, Dr. Scott Fishman, said. "What we didn't realize is that patients would use these drugs to opt out of life."

The "opioid crisis" is actually two separate crises, each with its own causes and solutions. One involves illegal narcotics, such as counterfeit fentanyl, and requires the attention of law enforcement as well as compassionate treatment for those addicted to these lethal drugs. The other crisis lies in the medical use of opioids, and its solution is much easier: Doctors need to use fewer opioids and turn to other ways of treating pain.

As for the Sacklers, they were now pariahs, the family's name stripped from the walls of museums and medical schools. Purdue Pharma filed for bankruptcy protection and, by 2021, the descendants of Mortimer and Raymond Sackler were offering to pay some $6 billion to buy protection for themselves from future lawsuits.

The Sacklers continued to insist that they had done nothing wrong and that critics were unfairly vilifying them. Still, during the years when they were making billions from OxyContin, the family apparently never sought to separate profits generated by legitimate prescriptions from those coming from prescriptions that ended up on the street.

It's possible that secret Purdue Pharma documents may emerge one day to show that the Sacklers really did try to sort out good money from bad. But if so, it's hard to understand why the family and their lawyers haven't publicized them.

The simple truth, it appears, is that all that money went into the same pot. That's how the OxyContin story began. And that is why it ended.

ACKNOWLEDGMENTS

OVER THE PAST TWO DECADES, COUNTLESS PEOPLE HAVE generously shared their insights, knowledge, and stories with me about the medical use of opioids and the opioid epidemic. But *Pain Killer* would never have been written without the participation and patience of Art Van Zee, Sue Ella Kobak, Jane Myers, Lindsay Myers, Russell Portenoy, Sister Beth Davies, Nathaniel Paul Katz, Jane Ballantyne, Larry Lavender, Laura Nagel, Gregory Wood, Terry Woodworth, and many other people. A number of former Purdue officials also shared their experiences with me, and I was grateful then and now for their leap of faith.

It is the rare author who gets to see a book reborn more than a decade after it went out of print. I now count myself among the lucky few. For that I owe a debt of gratitude to Hilary Redmond, my editor at Random House, whose enthusiasm for updating *Pain Killer* was infectious and whose ideas for how to reshape the book were invaluable. Everyone else at Random House, including Matthew Martin, Greg Kubie, Molly Turpin, and Evan Camfield, made my work easy. My thanks also go to Andrew Wylie and Kristina Moore at the Wylie Agency for finding such a good home for this new edition.

NOTES AND SOURCES

WHEN FIRST PUBLISHED IN 2003, THIS BOOK DREW ON MORE than two hundred interviews and a review of thousands of pages of documents including court records, internal Purdue documents, scientific reports, medical-journal articles, and newspaper and magazine articles.

My reporting about OxyContin started in 2001, with a series of articles I wrote for *The New York Times*. My interests soon expanded into associated areas I found fascinating, including the science of pain treatment, its history, and the growth of opioid use, as well as the history of drug advertising, prescription-drug abuse, and addiction.

In 2001, I visited Purdue headquarters, where I interviewed Michael Friedman, Howard Udell, and Paul Goldenheim for a *Times* article. I sought to interview them again when first writing this book, but they repeatedly declined to make themselves available or to respond to written questions.

In preparing this edition, I asked Purdue to point out any factual inaccuracies they believed were in the first edition so I could address them. The company chose not to respond. Michael Friedman and Paul Goldenheim also did not respond to inquiries. (Purdue's top lawyer, Howard Udell, died in 2013.)

1. Pill Hill

14 **by the following spring that figure had skyrocketed, in some areas to 90 percent:** Dennis Lee, Virginia Commonwealth attorney for Tazewell County, provided that estimate. Lee also said that forged $40 checks were so common that police officials joked, "We know where that forty dollars went."

16 **the company filed a required report:** Stravino's call to Purdue appears in an adverse-event action report filed by Purdue Pharma with the FDA.

17 **He picked up a copy of *The Boston Globe*:** Stravino read about OxyContin abuse in Washington County, Maine, in an article by Donna Gold in the *Globe* on May 21, 2000.

2. The War Against Pain

23 **80 percent of people:** The statistics on the unreliability of X-rays in the detection of back pain were cited by Dennis Turk in his paper "Clinicians' Attitudes about Prolonged Use of Opioids and the Issue of Patient Heterogeneity" in the *Journal of Pain and Symptom Management*, 1996.

24 **The history of pain management:** I have attempted only a brief and superficial accounting of the history of pain management and the medical science surrounding it. Along with Martin Booth's *Opium: A History*, books that may be of interest to the general reader are: *Why We Hurt: The Natural History of Pain* by Dr. Frank T. Vertosick Jr., and *The Culture of Pain* by David B. Morris.

24 **International Association for the Study of Pain:** It was Dr. John Bonica, a pain-management expert, who put together the 1973 meeting near Seattle that led to the formation a year later of the International Association for the Study of Pain. My very quick rendering of pain thought through the years is drawn from *Bonica's Management of Pain*, a textbook considered a bible for the field.

24 **doctors believed that opium was benign:** The descriptions of paregoric, laudanum, and Thomas Sydenham's comments are drawn from Martin Booth's *Opium*.

25 **"soldier's disease":** Civil War veterans were only one of the groups that included significant numbers of opiate addicts. According to historians like David Musto, white middle-class women represented another major one. Musto's book *The American Disease* (Yale University Press, 1973) is regarded as the classic text on the impact over the

years of government laws and regulations like the Harrison Act of 1914 on narcotics use, their abuse, and physician behavior.

26 **Dr. Saunders opened the first facility . . . in the final months of life:** Dr. Cicely Saunders was a remarkable woman. A nurse who cared for the dying in sterile hospital environments, she decided to go back to medical school to get a degree so that doctors would be forced to pay attention to her ideas. The first hospice in the United States opened in 1981 near New Haven, Connecticut.

27 **most notably Memorial Sloan Kettering:** While the movement to provide better cancer-pain care started in England, the cancer-pain researchers at Memorial Sloan Kettering prided themselves on taking a far more scientific approach than their British colleagues. They constantly ran tests on patients to determine which substances worked best. In the early 1980s, for example, Memorial Sloan Kettering was one of two hospitals that experimentally gave heroin to cancer patients while Congress debated whether to legalize its medical use. As it turned out, heroin, which is derived from morphine and breaks back down into it shortly after entering the body, wasn't any more effective.

28 **"chronic pain in litigation":** The description of the rapidly rising rate of back pain during the 1990s was cited in an article by Elisabeth Rosenthal in *The New York Times*, December 29, 1992. That same article also cited research by Dr. Michael Weintraub that had appeared in the *American Journal of Pain Management*, which looked at pain complaints by plaintiffs in lawsuits. It was Dr. Weintraub who said that patients may get subconsciously attached to pain because of financial rewards and suggested that "chronic pain in litigation" be viewed as a distinct syndrome.

28 **multidisciplinary approach to severe pain:** Descriptions of this approach were provided by Dr. Hubert L. Rosomoff, director of the Comprehensive Pain and Rehabilitation Center in Miami; Dennis Turk; and Barry Cole.

29 **"opiophobia":** The apparent origin of the term "opiophobia" is an article written by Dr. John P. Morgan in a 1986 issue of the journal *Controversies in Alcoholism and Substance Abuse*. Dr. Morgan's article was entitled "American Opiophobia: Customary Underutilization of Opioid Analgesics."

29 **Handing him a Bronx telephone book:** Russell Portenoy's 1986 study of drugstores was entitled "Unavailability of Narcotic Analgesics for Ambulatory Patients in New York City."

30 **a seminal figure . . . Dr. Kathleen M. Foley:** Along with her contributions to the field of cancer-pain treatment, Foley's advocacy efforts to improve the care of the terminally ill, a field known as palliative

care, were influential. She declined in 2003 to be interviewed for this book. Her observations and comments cited in this chapter are drawn from a 1996 oral history she gave for the John C. Liebeskind History of Pain Collection at UCLA. She was interviewed by Marcia L. Meldrum.

30 **in 1986 he published a study:** The report by Portenoy and Foley appeared in *Pain*.

32 **scientific holy trinity:** The three studies cited by Portenoy, pain-management activists, Purdue Pharma, and other drug companies in support of extremely minimal risk of iatrogenic addiction were "Drug Dependency in Patients with Chronic Headache," which appeared in *Headache* 17 (1977), 12–14; "Addiction Rare in Patients Treated with Narcotics," a letter in *The New England Journal of Medicine* 302 (1980), 123; and "Management of Pain during Debridement: A Survey of U.S. Burn Units," in *Pain* 13 (1982), 267–80.

36 **in a series of papers in the early 1990s:** David Joranson's writing on the issue of prescription-monitoring systems has appeared in a number of publications, including the *American Pain Society Bulletin* and the *Journal of Pharmaceutical Care in Pain & Symptom Control*. He declined to be interviewed in 2003 for this book.

38 **Purdue Pharma contributed half a million:** This contribution to the joint committee of the American Pain Society and the American Academy of Pain Management is found in a Purdue budget document.

38 **Drug companies also funded:** This information is drawn from documents obtained from the University of Wisconsin under that state's open-records law. They also show that Joranson served as a paid consultant to several opioid manufacturers, including Purdue.

3. Secrets of Dendur

42 **Dr. Arthur M. Sackler, sat before a panel of U.S. senators:** Sackler testified on January 30, 1962, before the subcommittee on antitrust and monopoly of the Senate Committee on the Judiciary.

44 **the company's sole shareholder was Else Sackler:** Medical & Science Communications Associates Inc. was originally known as Communications Associates. It changed its name on September 16, 1955, and a document associated with that name change identifies Else Sackler's role. A similarly named entity, Medical and Science Communications Development Corporation, operated as a holding company until Arthur Sackler's death. A 1968 stock certificate shows that

its stock was held in trust by Else Sackler, Mortimer Sackler, and Raymond Sackler, for the benefit of Carol Sackler, Arthur and Else's first child.

46 **Creedmoor State Hospital:** For more on the research work of Arthur, Mortimer, and Raymond Sackler, see *The New York Times*, November 2, 1951; September 8, 1957; and April 15, 1976.

47 **multipage color advertisement in . . . (*JAMA*):** Arthur Sackler was one of the original inductees in the Medical Advertising Hall of Fame. Some of his achievements are described in one of the group's publications, *Medicine Ave.* William G. Castagnoli was kind enough to provide me with a copy.

49 *The American Connection:* John Pekkanen's excellent book is a study of legislative battling and pharmaceutical-industry lobbying that shaped the Controlled Substances Act.

50 **Librium and Valium . . . he received bonus payments:** Michael Sonnenreich, Arthur Sackler's lawyer, told me this during an interview. I mentioned to him that I had heard that Sackler received a royalty based on each pill sold. He said that wasn't the case but explained that incentive bonuses were paid to Sackler when sales reached certain benchmarks.

51 **"happy baby vitamin":** The documents related to this bizarre episode are contained within the hearing record of the Kefauver committee.

52 **One favored vehicle . . . was the *Medical Tribune:*** For a quick flavor of the newspaper's slant, see Morton Mintz, *The Washington Post*, March 31, 1968.

52 **"Schizophrenics 'Wild'":** See Tamar Lewin, *The New York Times*, July 27, 1987.

53 **FDA officials investigated:** The comments about the article are drawn from a presentation by James C. Morrison, deputy director, Office of Drug Standards, on June 18, 1986.

53 **Mortimer and Raymond were fired:** See *The New York Times*, May 8, 1953.

54 **"When Spring Comes":** I found this advertising card on the Internet.

55 **Glutavite Corporation:** The company's original name was Medical Promotions Productions.

55 **John Lear:** His classic articles in *The Saturday Review* about the pharmaceutical industry should be required reading in every journalism and civics class. One benefit of working on this book was discovering them. For his reports related to the drug industry, the

FDA scandal, and the Sacklers, see *The Saturday Review*, January 3, 1959; February 7, 1959; June 4, 1960; July 2, 1960; March 3, 1962; and October 6, 1962.

60 **to avoid paying taxes:** Gertraud Sackler's claim was contained in a court filing in New York State Supreme Court.

63 **The ownership of MD Publications:** The precise transactions involving the ownership interests in MD Publications are not clear, but estate records indicate that a significant percentage of the company was owned at one point by Mortimer and Raymond Sackler or entities they controlled.

4. A Pot of Gold

64 **In the cover letter, a physician named Susan Bertrand:** Her letter was dated August 8, 2000.

64 **"Among the remedies which it has pleased":** Susan Bertrand's quotation from Thomas Sydenham, while accurate in spirit, may not have reflected a precise rendering of his words. In his exhaustive survey *Opium: A History* (St. Martin's Press, 1996), Martin Booth quoted Sydenham: "God, the giver of all good things, who hath granted to the human race, as a comfort in their afflictions, no medicine of the value of opium either in regard to the number of diseases it can control, or its efficiency in extirpating them."

66 **Van Zee had learned that the painkiller's abuse was occurring:** Newspapers that published articles in the spring and summer of 2000 about OxyContin abuse included the *Portland Press Herald*, *The Roanoke Times*, *The Columbus Dispatch*, and the *Anchorage Daily News*.

67 **"This probably will be your new Vicodin":** This quote from a law-enforcement official appeared in an article by Steve Cannizaro that appeared in *The Times-Picayune* on June 27, 2000.

68 **a Purdue physician, J. David Haddox:** Like other company executives, J. David Haddox declined to be interviewed in 2003 for this book. He also declined to provide a list of people familiar with his career. Several of those people, however, agreed to be interviewed.

69 **"pseudoaddiction":** The term was first used by Haddox and his co-author, Dr. David E. Weissman, in a paper titled "Opioid pseudoaddiction . . . an iatrogenic syndrome," *Pain*, 1989.

70 **a reporter at a small newspaper in southwestern Virginia:** Theresa M. Clemons was the reporter at the *Richlands News Press* who

was contacted by David Haddox. Her first article about the explosion of OxyContin abuse in Tazewell County appeared in the *News Press* on May 31, 2000. Haddox's quote regarding opioid addiction risks as being "one half of one percent" is from a follow-up article by Clemons that appeared on June 21, 2000.

71 **Purdue also knew that federal drug agents were investigating several doctors:** Mary Baluss, a pain-management advocate and lawyer in Washington, D.C., told me that several Purdue reps in Appalachia contacted her in mid-2000 and asked her to speak with physicians facing scrutiny over their prescribing. Baluss attended the Appalachian Pain Foundation's meeting in Richlands at the invitation of David Haddox, and on the way there she said they stopped off to see one of those physicians, Dr. Franklin Sutherland Jr. Not long afterward, Sutherland was indicted and convicted of illegally prescribing several drugs, including OxyContin.

71 **Purdue executives, working with Susan Bertrand:** Dr. Bertrand described the background of the Appalachian Pain Foundation during an interview I did with her in connection with an article for *The New York Times*.

76 **"Sounds like B.S. to me":** Diane Shnitzler's email to Curtis Wright was cited in the September 2006 prosecution memo sent to John Brownlee.

76 **"Actually, Diane, this is literally true":** Curtis Wright's email response to Diane Shnitzler was cited in the September 2006 prosecution memo.

76 **"so valuable and promotional":** Internal Purdue document cited in September 2006 prosecution memo.

77 **In one marketing document:** Each year Purdue produced a marketing document that laid out its plan, strategies, and budgets for the year ahead.

80 **"less than one percent":** This figure, which became Purdue's mantra in seeking to allay physician concerns of iatrogenic addiction, is repeatedly cited in company documents.

81 **"If I Only Had a Brain . . .":** This memo is dated November 4, 1996.

83 **One Myrtle Beach druggist:** I interviewed pharmacist Ron Mason while reporting an article for *The New York Times* about Comprehensive Care, the pain clinic there.

84 **Partners Against Pain:** Purdue's program was created in 1995.

5. Senior Night

87 **"a strategy to contain this!":** Robin Hogen's comment, written by hand on a copy of the warning sent by the U.S. Attorney in Maine to doctors, is cited in the September 2006 prosecution memo.

89 **a list of actions:** The list of proposed actions given by Art Van Zee to David Haddox was dated November 20, 2000.

92 **tiny town of St. Paul, Virginia:** The meeting at which Dr. David Fiellin and Dr. Richard Schottenfeld spoke took place on November 30, 2000.

93 **writing another letter:** The letter Art Van Zee sent to the FDA was dated December 3, 2000.

6. Hot Spots

97 **Sister Beth started the meeting:** The account of the town meeting at Lee High is drawn from an article that appeared in the *Powell Valley News*.

98 **a lengthy front-page article in *The New York Times*:** The article about "OxyFest" appeared on March 5, 2001. It was written by Melody Petersen and me.

102 **newspaper editorial boards to present their case:** A team of Purdue executives visited *The New York Times* in mid-2001 to complain about the paper's handling of the OxyContin story. Along with my articles, one by Paul Tough that appeared in the *Times Magazine* on July 29, 2001, had particularly incensed the company. At the meeting, the paper's editors said they believed that the coverage was fair. The company complained again about me in 2003 after the first edition of *Pain Killer* was published.

102 **a "new standard in corporate responsibility":** The comments of Purdue officials to the *Hartford Courant* were reported in *American Health Line*, July 19, 2001.

103 **"We were getting creamed":** Robin Hogen, Purdue's spokesman, made these comments during a 2002 conference held by Bulldog Reporter, an oddly named public-relations group. His talk was entitled "How to Respond When Your Product Comes Under Attack: OxyContin Fights Back."

106 **the local bank official who had come with them:** This man agreed to be interviewed on the condition that he not be identified.

107 **"I want to show you this":** Sister Beth Davies kept a copy of the ad prepared by Purdue.

7. Kiddie Dope

111 **Michael Friedman of Purdue quickly contacted Nagel:** His first letter to Nagel was dated March 8, 2001.

113 **"Purdue is working to gather":** Friedman's letter following up on Purdue's first meeting with Nagel was dated April 2, 2001.

116 **Florida officials announced . . . more overdose deaths from Oxy-Contin:** The data on Florida drug deaths was reported by Doris Bloodsworth in the *Orlando Sentinel*, May 27, 2001.

117 **Thomas Constantine:** The unhappiness of DEA agents with Mr. Constantine was reported by Gordon Wilkin in *U.S. News & World Report*, June 5, 1995.

118 **DEA announced:** The decision by the DEA to focus its efforts on OxyContin was reported in *The New York Times*, May 1, 2001.

119 **He also squared off against David Haddox:** Terry Woodworth and David Haddox debated each other on CBS's *Early Show*, May 3, 2001.

121 **"USA Today is planning an editorial":** Howard Udell's note to Laura Nagel was dated June 11, 2001; the paper's editorial appeared on June 13, 2001.

122 **Joranson's study:** David Joranson's study appeared in *JAMA* on April 5, 2000.

8. Purple Peelers

132 **the prestigious *Canadian Medical Association Journal*:** The study about the abuse of MS Contin was conducted by Dr. Amin Sajan, et al., of the University of British Columbia's Department of Family Practice. It and the accompanying editorial by Dr. Brian Goldman appeared in the *CMAJ* dated July 28, 1998.

135 **They arrested the clinic's operator, Dr. Frank Fisher:** The California state attorney general, Kamala Harris, announced the arrest of Dr. Fisher in February 1999.

136 **"Too much heroin and too many Oxycontins":** The article quoting

William Beatty was written by Linda Harris and appeared in *The Weirton Daily Times* on April 20, 1999.

136 **a Purdue sales rep in western Pennsylvania:** The warning to doctors in Cambria County, Pennsylvania, about the growing abuse of OxyContin was sent on August 5, 1999. Ron Portash, the law-enforcement official who wrote it, told me that he included other drugs besides OxyContin to focus "not solely on OxyContin, and at that time risk a lawsuit from the pharmaceutical industry."

137 **Leon V. Dulion:** The Purdue sales rep gave that testimony in October 1999 during a pre-trial deposition in the case of Dr. James Graves.

138 **All felony charges against him:** In 2004, Dr. Frank Fisher was also acquitted after a trial of the remaining misdemeanor charges against him.

9. The Body Count

141 **McCloskey vehemently disputed:** Interview with Jay McCloskey.

144 **$10,000:** In October 2002, Purdue's political-action committee made two $5,000 donations to Senator Christopher Dodd, campaign finance records show.

145 **"our company looked like food":** Hogen's comments are from his 2002 speech before the public-relations group Bulldog Reporter.

145 **Rudolph W. Giuliani:** He declined through a spokesperson to be interviewed for this book when first published.

146 **"The mayor and I just met with Asa Hutchinson":** Bernard Kerik's comments were reported by Chris Smith in *New York* magazine, September 15, 2002.

149 **"We don't believe there is cause for panic":** See *The New York Times*, April 15, 2002.

150 **Butterworth's inquiry:** Several reporters, including myself, petitioned to receive the file of Bob Butterworth's investigation into Purdue under Florida's open-records law. Purdue sought to block the release of those records but lost in court. The file contained, among other documents, the company's marketing budget plans for the years 1996 to 2002; notes from the interview with William Gergely, a former Purdue rep; and the letters between Jody Collins and a Purdue lawyer.

10. A Reckoning

157   **Dr. Nathaniel Paul Katz:** Nat Katz was a generous guide for me to the field of pain treatment and opioids.

158   **A doctor from Indiana:** Dr. Stephen Baker's grand-jury testimony is cited in the September 2006 prosecution memo.

158   **Mark Ross:** His testimony is cited in the September 2006 prosecution memo. In it, he describes giving doctors Dr. Daniel Brookoff's 1993 study about the lack of appeal of time-release opioids to drug abusers.

160   **a Purdue-funded study:** The study was known informally as the "Roth report." It was conducted by Dr. Sanford Roth and published in the *Archives of Internal Medicine* on June 26, 2000, as "Around the Clock, Controlled Release Oxycodone Use in Osteoarthritis."

160   **"Howard, Michael, and Paul agree":** This email, concerning the continuing distribution of the Roth study, was written in August 2003 and was cited in the September 2006 prosecutors' memo.

162   **Sara was hardly an ideal witness:** Interview with Paul Hanly.

162   **she sent Udell an email:** Maureen Sara's email to Howard Udell is cited in the prosecutors' memo.

162   **testimony by Sara in a deposition:** Her deposition testimony is cited in the prosecutors' memo. The deposition was sealed and it is not known if Sara was questioned by Purdue lawyers. Her lawsuit against Purdue was dismissed, according to Paul Hanly.

163   **the three men be indicted:** In their memo, prosecutors said they were prepared to bring several charges against Friedman, Udell, and Goldenheim, including conspiracy to defraud the United States and related charges including mail fraud, wire fraud, misbranding of a drug, and money laundering. Prosecutors also wrote they were prepared to charge Goldenheim with making false statements before Congress. The specific felony charges recommended by prosecutors and one document cited in their memo were first reported by Katherine Eban in *Fortune*, "OxyContin: Purdue Pharma's Painful Medicine," November 9, 2011.

164   **an eight-hour presentation:** Two lawyers present at the meeting described it.

165   **anticipated that defense lawyers:** In their prosecution memo, government lawyers described the anticipated defenses that Purdue and its executives would raise.

165   **Alice S. Fisher:** Fisher left the Justice Department in 2008 and is now in private practice. She did not respond to emails seeking to set

up an interview about her reported role in rejecting felony charges against Purdue's executives. Two lawyers present at the October 11, 2006, meeting said Fisher was in attendance.

167 **a history that would bar them:** Michael Friedman, Howard Udell, and Paul Goldenheim repeatedly made administrative and legal appeals to overturn their disbarment from holding executive positions with drug companies doing business with the government. They were unsuccessful but got the length of their disbarment reduced from twenty years to twelve years. In one appeal, they argued in 2010 to federal judge Ellen Segal Huvelle that their convictions were solely a reflection of their senior status at Purdue. "Plaintiffs seem to misunderstand or misstate the basic elements of the conviction," Judge Huvelle wrote. (Howard Udell died in 2013, at age seventy-two. In 2009, he founded the Connecticut Veterans Legal Center, which provided free legal advice to veterans.)

171 **In his response, the prosecutor said:** John Brownlee testified before the Senate Judiciary Committee on July 31, 2007, at a hearing entitled "Evaluating the Propriety and Adequacy of the OxyContin Criminal Settlement." He was also asked at the hearing about the circumstances that transpired after he received a telephone call from Paul McNulty's aide, Michael Elston, asking him to slow down resolution of the Purdue case. At the time of the call, then–U.S. Attorney General Alberto Gonzales was dismissing U.S. Attorneys in hat critics called politically motivated firings. Eight days after Brownlee Elston's request, his name was placed on the firing list. However, Brownlee was not fired.

11. Empire of Deceit

174 *Esquire* **magazine:** Christopher Glazek's article, "The Secretive Family Making Billions from the Opioid Crisis," appeared on October 16, 2017.

174 *The New Yorker:* Patrick Radden Keefe's article, "The Family That Built an Empire of Pain," appeared on October 30, 2017.

174 **"morally abhorrent to me":** Elizabeth Sackler's comments were made in an article published in *The New York Times* on January 22, 2018.

175 **a newspaper there reported:** That newspaper was the *Charleston Gazette-Mail*. The reporter who wrote the articles, Eric Eyre, won the 2017 Pulitzer Prize for Investigative Reporting. Shortly afterward, the newspaper filed for bankruptcy.

175   **drug-industry lobbyists succeeded:** See *The Washington Post*, October 15, 2017.

177   **"Recovery of Morphine from a Controlled Release Preparation":** The article sent to Richard Sackler and Howard Udell appeared in the December 15, 1990, issue of the journal *Cancer*, according to the prosecution memo.

178   **that researcher wrote:** According to the prosecution memo, Purdue researcher Gary Richie was assigned to review how abusers were extracting morphine from MS Contin and a competing drug, Oramorph.

178   **an American medical publication:** According to the prosecution memo, a subordinate sent Paul Goldenheim a copy of a publication called *American Family Physician*.

178   **drug addicts in New Zealand:** Dr. Robert Kaiko, a top Purdue scientist, sent an email in March 2007 to Mortimer Sackler and other Purdue executives stating that "MST [MS Contin's brand name outside the U.S.] is the most common sources [sic] of paternally abused morphine/heroin," the prosecution memo states.

178   **"We do not have a postmarketing abuse monitoring system":** Dr. Robert Kaiko made that statement in the same March 2007 email in which he discussed MS Contin abuse in New Zealand, according to the prosecution memo.

178   **a legal memo entitled "MS Contin Abuse":** Udell sent his memo describing newspaper reports of OxyContin abuse in Canada on March 19, 1998, to Mortimer Sackler, Raymond Sackler, Richard Sackler, Kathe Sackler, Jonathan Sackler, Samantha S. Sackler, and Mortimer D. A. Sackler, the prosecution memo states.

179   **"was enough to keep a person busy all day":** The email by Mark Alfonso citing discussions of OxyContin abuse in chat rooms was sent on October 3, 1997, to James J. Lang, a Purdue vice president and marketing official, and copied to Michael Friedman, the prosecution memo stated.

180   **Howard Udell alerted a fellow company executive:** Udell's comment was contained in a legal memorandum he sent on December 10, 1998, to John Stewart, the head of Purdue's operation in Canada, the prosecution memo states. In it, Udell also thanked Stewart for sending the company the *Canadian Medical Association Journal* study. Stewart, who served as chief executive of Purdue from 2007 to 2013, is reportedly now in the marijuana business.

180   **During a two-week period in August 1999:** These episodes of OxyContin abuse and associated crimes are recounted in the prosecution memo.

181   **memo sent by a Purdue district manager:** The memo was sent by
       a sales manager, Mark Radcliffe, on November 18, 1999, the prose-
       cution memo states.

182   **"I simply do not want us to over-react":** The email exchange be-
       tween David Haddox and Michael Friedman and other Purdue ex-
       ecutives about Haddox's suggestion for a crisis-response plan took
       place between November 30 and December 8, 1999, according to the
       prosecution memo.

182   **117 call reports:** All the states where the terms "street value,"
       "crush," or "snort" were found in call notes were listed in the prose-
       cution memo.

183   **"I recall that I received this kind of news on MS Contin":** Mark
       Alfonso's email recounting his recollections of significant MS
       Contin–related abuse was sent to Robin Hogen on June 19, 2000,
       and copied to Michael Friedman, the prosecution memo states.

183   **"all this chat on e-mail?":** In forwarding Alfonso's email, Friedman
       asked Udell that question, the prosecution memo states.

183   **The scope of the profits:** The annual sales of MS Contin and Oxy-
       Contin are cited in the prosecution memo, as is the manner of
       awarding bonuses based on those sales. In addition, the prosecution
       memo provided details about the network of corporate entities used
       by Raymond and Mortimer Sackler.

184   **a March 2001 telephone-answering-machine message:** Robin
       Hogen left his message on March 15, 2001, according to the prosecu-
       tion memo.

Epilogue: The War Against Pain Revisited

190   **a little-noticed study:** Dr. Jane Ballantyne's study, entitled "Opioid
       Therapy for Chronic Pain," was published in *The New England Jour-
       nal of Medicine* on November 13, 2003.

191   **Denmark:** Unlike the United States, countries such as Denmark
       with socialized-medicine systems have long had computerized medi-
       cal records that researchers can use to track treatments and patients'
       outcomes. A Danish pain expert, Per Sjögren, looked at relative re-
       covery times of those treated with opioids and other methods.

191   **Department of Veterans Affairs:** The VA has come under much-
       deserved criticism for its overuse of opioids and other powerful med-
       ications in treating military personnel, particularly those returned
       from deployments to Iraq and Afghanistan. More recently, however,

the VA system has been in the forefront of researching alternative means of treating pain and utilizing those techniques in practice.

191 **"Addiction is not the real problem":** Dr. Scott Fishman's comments appeared in an e-book I wrote called *A World of Hurt*, which was published by *The New York Times* in 2013.

INDEX

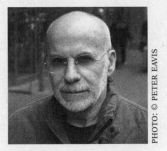

BARRY MEIER worked for nearly three decades as a reporter for *The New York Times* and was a member of the *Times* team that won the 2017 Pulitzer Prize for International Reporting. He is also a two-time winner of the prestigious George Polk Award and other honors. He was the first journalist to shed a national spotlight on the abuse of OxyContin and also exposed the dangers of various drugs and medical products, including a defective heart device and a generation of flawed artificial hips. Prior to the *Times*, he worked at *The Wall Street Journal* and *New York Newsday*.

Meier is the author of *Missing Man* and *Spooked*. He lives in New York.

barrymeierbooks.com
Facebook.com/barry.meier1
Twitter: @BarryMeier